An Introduction to Cell and Tissue Transplantation Science

British Blood Transfusion Society
and
British Association for Tissue Banking

Editors:
Andrew Hadley
Helen Gillan
James Foreman

© Second Edition: November 2011

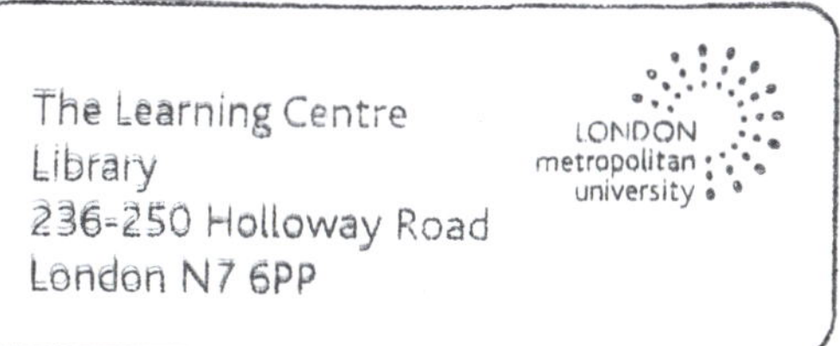

CONTRIBUTORS

Prof John Armitage
Director of Tissue Banking, Bristol Eye Hospital.

Dr Eric Austin
Laboratory Director, Stem Cell and Immunotherapies, NHSBT

Mr Kyle Bennett
Tissue Bank Manager, Tissue Services, NHSBT

Dr Akila Chandrasekhar
Consultant, Tissue Services, NHSBT

Mr James Foreman
BATB

Dr George Galea
National Tissue Services Director, SNBTS

Helen Gillan
Head of Operations – Tissue Services, NHSBT

Dr Martin Guttridge
Laboratory Director, Stem Cell and Immunotherapies, NHSBT &
Manager NHS Cord Blood Bank, NHSBT

Dr Andrew Hadley
General Manager, Specialist Services Operations, NHSBT

Dr Bing Jones
Associate Specialist, Sheffield, NHSBT

Prof John Kearney
Head of Tissue Services / Assistant Director, Clinical Science, NHSBT

Dr Richard Lomas
Senior Clinical Development Manager, Tissue Services, NHSBT

Dr Anatole Lubenko
Laboratory Director, Stem Cell and Immunotherapies, NHSBT

Dr Cristina Navarrete
National Head, Histocompatibility & Immunogenetics, NHSBT

Dr Derwood Pamphilon
Consultant Haematologist, NHSBT

Mr Robert Parker
Head of Heart Valve Bank, Royal Brompton Hospital

Prof David Pegg
Professor of Cryobiology, University of York

Amanda Ranson
Regional Tissue Donation Manager, NHSBT

Dr Paul Rooney
R&D Manager, Tissue Services, NHSBT

Dr Ann Smith
Head of Stem Cell Transplant Laboratory, Royal Marsden NHS Foundation Trust

2

Prof Suzanne Watt
National Head, Stem Cell and Immunotherapies, NHSBT

Dr Claire Wiggins
Laboratory Director, Stem Cell and Immunotherapies, NHSBT

CONTENTS

TISSUE TRANSPLANTATION SCIENCE 155

19 COLLECTION AND RETRIEVAL OF TISSUE 156

20 TISSUE PROCESSING, STORAGE AND ISSUE 170

1 FORWARD TO 2ND EDITION

The first edition of this book was published in 2007 to provide a core text for healthcare professionals working in tissue banks and stem cell laboratories. This second edition reflects advances in clinical practice as well as comments and suggestions received following publication of edition 1.

Advances captured in this edition include developments in the use of cord blood for stem cell transplantation, transfusion support for transplant patients and a re-appraisal of the regulatory environment for cell and tissue transplantation.

The first section of the book covers core topics such as the biology of stem cells and tissues as well as subjects common to both stem cells and tissues including regulation. There are two further sections covering stem cell transplantation science and tissue transplantation science.

Candidates are reminded that the content of this text book must be supplemented with additional reading and research in order to successfully pass the specialist certificate examination.

The editors are especially grateful to Ann Smith, Bob Parker, Claire Wiggins, George Galea, Cristina Navarrete and Lorraine Tresnak for their contributions to edition two.

Andrew Hadley, Helen Gillan and James Foreman

2 INTRODUCTION

2.1 The BBTS/BATB Specialist Certificate in Cell and Tissue Transplantation Science

This book aims to provide the basic information required by healthcare professionals working in laboratories supporting cell and tissue transplantation. It is intended as a core text for staff working towards the BBTS/BATB Specialist Certificate in Cell and Tissue Transplantation Science.

The British Blood Transfusion Society (BBTS) and the British Association for Tissue Banking (BATB) are committed to supporting training and education. The BBTS and BATB have noted the common competencies required by staff working in tissue banks and laboratories supporting stem cells transplantation. These activities are governed by EU and UK legislation requiring systems of continuous professional development (CPD) for staff. As such, this training is aimed at UK Health Professions Council (HPC) registered scientists who are looking to specialise in Cell and Tissue Transplantation Science.

While this book provides some of the basic factual information required at Healthcare Scientist Career Stage 6, it is _essential_ that students seeking to take the BBTS/BATB Specialist Certificate examination supplement this information by referring to textbooks, reviews, guidelines and web sites. Relevant material is referenced throughout this book. The information provided within this book is intended for use in conjunction with in-service practical training.

An explanation of abbreviations and terminology used throughout this book is provided at Chapter 24.

2.2 Questions and Answers

At the end of each section of this book there are a number of questions for you to answer. To make best use of the book, read each section in turn, answering the questions in writing before looking at the answers which can be found at the back of the book. It is recommended that other references identified within each section are also read. If you have not understood something, you should re-read the section and/or refer to one of the recommended text books.

2.3 Assignments and Scenarios

Throughout this book there are assignments intended to help you develop your knowledge by providing a focus for further reading and study. These assignments are not intended to be optional; rather they seek to help candidates develop a level of core knowledge consistent with 'Specialist Certificate' level. This book does not provide 'answers' for assignments; you are advised to share your written assignment work with a work place supervisor or mentor (see below) in order to receive constructive feedback and comment.

The examination process for BBTS/BATB Specialist Certificate includes an assessment of the candidate's ability to apply knowledge in various problem-solving scenarios. These scenarios will test the candidate's ability to draw on knowledge and experience from a range of sources.

Candidates are strongly encouraged to discuss 'real-life' situations as they arise from time to time in their workplace with their line manager or mentor, considering carefully how scientific, clinical, regulatory and technical knowledge should be applied in each situation.

2.4   Mentors

It is strongly recommended that candidates intending to sit the BBTS/BATB Specialist Certificate examination identify a mentor to provide guidance, advice and encouragement throughout the period of study. A work place supervisor or line manager would usually fulfil this role. The BBTS and/or BATB may be able to assist candidates where a suitable mentor is not available within the workplace.

2.5   Training to SOPs and Maintaining Records

The training identified within this book is additional to Standard Operating Procedure (SOP) training. SOPs are detailed step-by-step accounts of how procedures must be carried out. They are used to maintain a consistent performance from operator to operator, and to ensure that the same standards are continually applied over an extended period. They are also used to train operators to a consistent standard and trainers should ensure that the person being trained has a good understanding of an SOP and can apply it in practice.

CORE SUBJECTS

3   THE REGULATION OF CELL AND TISSUE BANKING

3.1   Introduction

The regulatory framework for cell and tissue banking has evolved over a number of years. The procurement of tissues from deceased donors has been controlled via UK law since the 1960s (Human Tissue Act 1961). In 1992 the British Association for Tissue Banking was formed by like minded tissue banking professionals who realised that as a collective they were better able to increase standards within the profession and lobby government for stricter legislation.

It was not until 2001 that the Department of Health issued the *Code of Practice for Tissue Banks*. This was a voluntary code which described the quality system required and also the acceptable standard of facility required by a Tissue Bank. The Code of Practice for Tissue Banks applied to Cell, Tissue and Cord Blood Banks. It was inspected by the Medicines and Healthcare products Regulatory Authority (MHRA). The MHRA are the inspectorate for the *Rules and Guidelines for the Manufacturers and Distributors of Pharmaceuticals* (also known as the "Orange Guide"). This guide sets out the requirements of "Good Manufacturing Practice" (GMP). Although parts of GMP are not relevant to cell and tissue banking, the principles and techniques of GMP form the backbone of all current regulations and quality system requirements. The Code of Practice for Tissue Banks remained current until the *European Tissue and Cells Directive* and changes to UK Law updated the regulatory climate for tissue and cell banking in 2006.

3.2   Human Tissue Act 2004

Following several high profile tissue and organ retention stories (Bristol Royal Infirmary, Alder Hey Children's Hospital) the law regulating human tissue was overhauled. The Human Tissue Act 2004 (HT Act) repeals and replaces the Human Tissue Act 1961, Anatomy Act 1984 and the Human Organ Transplants Act 1989 for England and Wales. There is a separate HT (Scotland) Act which requires authorisation rather than consent.

The HT Act requires consent for the storage and use of tissues and cells from the living or deceased for specific health related purposes. It defines the "scheduled purposes" for which consent is required. The HT Act regulates the removal, storage and use of human tissue including human cells. It came into force on 1st September 2006.

The HT Act named the "Human Tissue Authority" as the competent authority under the EUTCD for the regulation of tissue and cells. The Human Fertilisation and Embryology Authority (HFEA) are the competent authority under the EUTCD for the regulation of gametes and embryos for human application.

3.3 European Tissue and Cells Directive (EUTCD)

The aim of the EUTCD is to harmonise standards in cell and tissue banking to protect the safety of recipients of cells and tissues across the European Union. The EUTCD is made up of three Directives, the parent Directive (2004/23/EC) which provides the framework legislation and two technical directives (2006/17/EC and 2006/86/EC), which provide the detailed requirements of the EUTCD. The Directive sets out minimum standards for activities relating to cells and tissues for human application. This includes the traceability of tissue and cells from donor to recipient. The EUTCD also mandates member states to devise systems for the reporting of adverse events and to report annual activity data from the tissue establishments.

3.4 Human Tissue (Quality and Safety for Human Application) Regulations 2007

The Directives were fully implemented into UK Law on 5th July 2007 via the *Human Tissue (Quality and Safety for Human Application) Regulations 2007* (Q&S Regulations).

This expanded the remit of the HTA to include the regulation of:
- Procurement
- Testing
- Processing
- Storage
- Distribution
- Import and export of tissues and cells for human application.

A Tissue Bank undertaking any of the above activities is required to apply for a licence under the Q&S Regulations.

3.5 HTA Directions

The HTA issues Directions for licensed tissue establishments to take into account changes to policy and legislation. Examples:

HTA Directions 002/2009

Directions bringing into force HTA codes of practice. These Directions
revoke Directions 002/2006

HTA Directions 001/2010

Directions bringing into force annual compliance reporting for establishments with an HTA post mortem licence.

HTA Directions 002/2010

Directions bringing into force an audit of relevant material removed from deceased persons during post-mortem examination, for establishments with an HTA post mortem licence.

HTA Directions 003/2010

The Directions consolidate and clarify the standards required under the Human Tissue (Quality and Safety of Tissues and Cells for Human Application) Regulations 2007. These Directions revoke Directions 001/2006, 002/2007 and 004/2007

3.5.1   Human Tissue Authority

The HTA "license and inspect organisations that store and use human tissue for purposes such as research, patient treatment, post-mortem examination, teaching and public exhibitions." They also "give approval for organ and bone marrow donations from living people."

Further information about the other sectors (apart from human application) that the HTA regulate can be found on the HTA website (www.hta.gov.uk).

3.5.2   Licensing

Tissue Establishments were required to apply for a license for storage of tissue for human application by 7th April 2006. A licence for all other activities was required from 1st September 2006. The licence is under the Quality and Safety Regulations and includes procurement, testing, processing, storage, import /export and distribution of tissues and/or cells for human application.

A licence is required for storage of tissue / cells intended for human application for more than 48 hours. The tissue / cells have to be classified as a "relevant material" under the HT Act. For the purposes of the HT Act, a "relevant material" means material other than gametes which consists of or includes human cells.

The application process is via an on-line compliance report and should be completed by the Licence Holder and Designated Individual for the tissue establishment.

Several roles are defined on the licence:

Licence Holder ~ is normally a corporate body that has a duty to ensure that the conditions of third part agreements are complied with, that Directions are complied with and that fees are paid.

Designated Individual ~ is the person supervising the licensed activity and has several responsibilities including ensuring that suitable practices are used in undertaking the licensed activity and that other persons who work under the licence are suitable. He/She must be appropriately qualified e.g. have evidence of a formal qualification in the medical or biological sciences or be considered by the HTA as suitably qualified and have at least 2 years practical experience which is directly relevant to the licensed activity.

Person Designated ~ these are the responsible members of staff on site (e.g. Tissue Bank Manager, Stem Cell Bank Manager, Quality Manager)

3.5.3   Inspection

The HTA has two phases of inspection. The first phase is the analysis of the compliance report licence application. A decision is made on whether to grant a licence, grant a licence with additional conditions, or refuse a licence.

          17

The second phase of inspection is the site visit. This is normally a pre-arranged visit to the tissue establishment although the HTA can perform unannounced site inspection visits.

The second phase inspection is planned to assess the facilities, methods and personnel to ensure that they meet the requirements of the Tissue Quality and Safety Regulations 2007. Following an inspection visit additional conditions which are time limited can be added to a licence to ensure that required improvements are implemented. Other regulatory action may be instigated including the suspension or revocation of the licence.

The HTA also has a statutory duty to provide advice and guidance to tissue establishments.

The HTA has published Codes of Practice which are brought into force via Directions. These include:

Code of Practice 1: Consent,

Code of Practice 2: Donation of organs, tissue and cells for transplantation

Code of Practice 5: Removal, storage and disposal of human organs and tissue

Code of Practice 6: Donation of allogeneic bone marrow and peripheral blood stem cells for transplantation

Full, up to date versions of these codes are available on the HTA website. (www.hta.gov.uk)

3.5.4 Third Party Agreements

Any "third party" performing a licensed activity on behalf of a licensed tissue establishment must do so under a "third party agreement" e.g. storage, testing etc.

3.5.5 Satellite Sites

If the licensed tissue establishment operates over a number of sites then there will be a licensed "hub" tissue establishments linked to "satellite sites". The "satellite sites" must operate with the same standard operating procedures and must be under the direction of the Designated Individual.

3.5.6 Adverse Event Reporting

Under the EUTCD the HTA is required to operate a system for tissue establishments to report serious adverse events and reactions. The HTA then has a responsibility to trend and investigate events to ensure that they have been appropriately reported, investigated and actioned.

The definitions from the EUTCD are:

"Serious Adverse Event (SAE)

'serious adverse event' means any untoward occurrence associated with the procurement, testing, processing, storage and distribution of tissues and cells that might lead to the transmission of a communicable disease, to death or life-threatening, disabling or incapacitating conditions for patients or which might result in, or prolong, hospitalisation or morbidity.

Serious Adverse Reaction (SAR)

'serious adverse reaction' means an unintended response, including a communicable disease, in the donor or in the recipient associated with the procurement or human application of tissues and cells that is fatal, life threatening, disabling, incapacitating or which results in, or prolongs, hospitalisation or morbidity."

3.5.7 Annual Activity Reporting

The HTA is also tasked with reporting to the European Union on activity in all tissue establishments. This is reported in January each year and includes all licensed activity undertaken in the previous calendar year.

3.5.8 European Coding System

Under the EUTCD, a Europe wide coding system for the traceability of human tissue and cells must be established. The system which has been chosen is ISBT 128. This is in the early stages of implementation.

3.6   Other Relevant Regulations

3.6.1 Standards for HPC Collection, Processing and Transplantation

These standards were drawn up by the Joint Accreditation Committee of ISCT-Europe and EBMT (European Group for Blood and Marrow Transplantation) and are referred to as JACIE. They are written specifically for stem cell transplantation. They are designed to provide minimum standards for facilities and individuals performing haematopoietic cell transplantation and therapy or providing support services for such procedures. Governmental laws or regulations may establish additional requirements.

3.6.2 Guidelines for the Blood Transfusion Services in the UK (Red Book)

The *Guidelines for the Blood Transfusion Services in the United Kingdom* or "Red Book" as it is more commonly referred to, were first published in 1990 by HMSO. They were first compiled by experts from the Regional Transfusion Centres and the National Institute of Biological Standards and Control (NIBSC) and aimed to define guidelines for all materials produced by the UK Blood Transfusion Services for both therapeutic and diagnostic use. As the services, provided by the UK Blood Transfusion Services has expanded to include processing and storage of tissues and human progenitor cells the guidelines have been expanded to include guidelines for these processes and products.

The *Red Book* is now compiled by a group of experts involving many from outside of blood transfusion services, now called the Joint UKBTS/NIBSC Professional Advisory Committee (JPAC) through Standing Advisory Committees (SACs) representing the various disciplines within the Blood Transfusion Services.

3.6.3   FACT-NETCORD

NETCORD was formally established in 1997 and is now recognised as the largest source of cord blood grafts for patients in need of haematopoietic stem cells transplantation. The affiliated cord blood banks, throughout the world, provide units of cord blood of varied ethnicity for transplant. In co-operation with the Foundation for Accreditation of Cellular Therapy (FACT), NETCORD developed international standards for cord blood banks. Individual banks, world-wide, use these standards to achieve excellence in their procedures and products and many have applied for FACT-NETCORD accreditation.

3.6.4   Quality Management System Fundamentals

Regardless of the regulatory framework which defines the requirements of a particular sector, the fundamentals of the quality management systems are the same. The regulations define the standards required for processing, air quality etc but without the overarching quality system there is no process for ensuring that the quality of the tissue and cells are controlled and meet the safety and efficacy required for the protection of patients.

This section defines the fundamentals required:

Quality System:

The quality system must be defined and documented.

Document control:

A defined system of ensuring that all documents are approved by an appropriate person, version controlled to prevent obsolete versions being available, archived to ensure the document history is preserved and validated to ensure that the procedure describes the process adequately.

Traceability:

All products must be traceable from donor to recipient. This includes all consumables.

Personnel:

All personnel must have their roles and responsibilities adequately defined. They must be competent in their roles and understand their responsibilities. The competency and training must be documented.

Premises and Equipment:

All facilities and equipment must be fit for purpose. They must be validated prior to use to ensure that they meet the requirements of the process.

Adverse Events / Quality Incidents:

Non-conforming product or process must be recorded and root cause analysis performed. Corrective action must be implemented to prevent the non-conformance occurring again.

Self-inspection / Audit:

Activities within the establishment must be regularly independently audited to ensure compliance with the quality system.

3.7   Appropriate Consent

The Human Tissue Act 2004 (which extends to England, Wales and Northern Ireland) sets out a legal framework for the storage and use of tissue from the living and for the removal, storage and use of tissue and organs from the dead. This includes 'residual' tissue following clinical and diagnostic procedures. These activities carry a statutory requirement for consent.

3.7.1   Living donors

Consent for treatment and examination including removal is a matter for criminal law. Under the Human Tissue Act, tissue may be taken in a variety of circumstances. For example:

- in the course of diagnostic procedures, e.g., taking a blood or urine sample, tissue biopsy, cervical screening;

- in the course of a treatment procedure, e.g., removing tissue (organs, tumours, etc.) during surgery;

- when removed specifically for the purpose of research.

Once tissue has been taken from patients, for whatever purpose, it can be stored and used without consent for a number of purposes.

Consent from the living is needed for storage and use of tissue for:

- Obtaining scientific or medical information which may be relevant to any other person, now or in the future;

- Research in connection with disorders, or the functioning, of the human body;

- Public display;

- Transplantation.

Consent from the living is <u>not</u> needed for storage and use of tissue for:

- clinical audit;

- Education or training relating to human health (including training for research into disorders, or the functioning, of the human body);

- Performance assessment;

- Public health monitoring.

- Quality assurance.

3.7.2   The Deceased

Consent is needed for the removal, storage and use of tissue from deceased donors for the following scheduled purposes:

- Anatomical examination;

- Determining the cause of death;

- Obtaining scientific or medical information, which may be relevant to any other person now or in the future;

- Public display;

- Research in connection with disorders, or the functioning, of the human body;

- Transplantation;

- Clinical audit;

- Education or training relating to human health;

- Performance assessment;

- Public health monitoring;

- Quality assurance.

3.7.3   Some Exceptions

Tissue from living individuals may be stored for use and/or used without consent, provided that:

- The research is ethically approved;

  and

- The tissue is anonymised such that the researcher is not in possession of information identifying the person from whose body the material has come and is not likely to come into possession of it.

3.7.4   Giving Consent

For consent to be valid it must be given voluntarily by an appropriately informed person who has the capacity to agree to the activity in question. If an adult is competent, only they are permitted to give consent.

The Human Tissue Act allows residual tissue samples left over following a diagnostic or therapeutic intervention or research to be disposed of lawfully. However, residual tissue is often an important source of material for research, and surgical consent forms may include an agreement to the use of such tissue for purposes such as research, education and training.

Adults are said to be competent to consent if they can understand the nature and purpose of the proposed procedure, understand and retain information relevant to the decision, and weigh the necessary information to arrive at a choice.

Under the Act, a child is defined as being under 18 years old. Children may consent to a proposed medical procedure or the storage and use of their tissue if they are competent to do so. A child is considered to be competent to give valid consent to a proposed intervention if they have sufficient intelligence and understanding to enable them fully to understand what is involved. A person who has parental responsibility for the child can consent on his/her behalf only if the child has not made a decision and is not competent to do so or chooses not to make that decision (although competent to do so).

Where an adult has, whilst alive and competent, given consent for one or more of the scheduled purposes to take place following their death, then that consent is sufficient for the activity to be lawful.

If a deceased adult has neither consented to nor specifically refused any particular donation those close to them should be asked whether a nominated representative was appointed to take those decisions. The nominated representative can consent to the removal, storage and use of tissue. If the deceased person has neither indicated their consent nor nominated representative, then the appropriate consent can be given by someone in a 'qualifying relationship' to the deceased. Those in a qualifying relationship to the deceased person are (highest first):

- spouse or partner

- parent or child

- brother or sister

3.7.5   Codes of Practice

The HTA has produced a series of 'Codes of Practice' covering consenting and related issues in detail, including the donation of allogeneic stem cells. These Codes are referenced below.

- Code of practice 1 - Consent -
  http://www.hta.gov.uk/legislationpoliciesandcodesofpractice/codesofpractice/code1consent.cfm

- Code of practice 2 - Donation of solid organs for transplantation -
  http://www.hta.gov.uk/legislationpoliciesandcodesofpractice/codesofpractice/code2donationoforgans.cfm

- Code of practice 3 - Post-mortem examination -
  http://www.hta.gov.uk/legislationpoliciesandcodesofpractice/codesofpractice/code3post-mortem.cfm

- Code of practice 4 - Anatomical examination -
  http://www.hta.gov.uk/legislationpoliciesandcodesofpractice/codesofpractice/code4anatomy.cfm

- Code of practice 5 - Disposal of human tissue -
  http://www.hta.gov.uk/legislationpoliciesandcodesofpractice/codesofpractice/code5disposal.cfm

PLEASE NOTE: the HTA has provided further clarification on the disposal of identifiable material and paragraph 73 in this code has been amended. This code does not require Parliamentary approval to have effect, so can be amended by the HTA as it feels appropriate.

- Code of practice 6 - Donation of allogeneic bone marrow and peripheral blood stem cells for transplantation - http://www.hta.gov.uk/legislationpoliciesandcodesofpractice/codesofpractice/code6 donationofbonemarrow.cfm

- Code of practice 7 - Public display - http://www.hta.gov.uk/legislationpoliciesandcodesofpractice/codesofpractice/code7 publicdisplay.cfm

- Code of practice 8 - Import and export of human bodies, body parts and tissue - http://www.hta.gov.uk/legislationpoliciesandcodesofpractice/codesofpractice/code8i mportandexport.cfm

PLEASE NOTE: code of practice 8 was published in May 2007 and has not been revised.

- Code of practice 9 - Research - http://www.hta.gov.uk/legislationpoliciesandcodesofpractice/codesofpractice/code9r esearch.cfm

3.8   Reading Material

1. Rules and Guidance for Pharmaceutical Manufacturers and Distributors (2007). http://www.mhra.gov.uk/Publications/Regulatoryguidance/Medicines/CON203022 91
2. Guidelines for the Blood Transfusion Services in the UK (7th edition). http://www.transfusionguidelines.org.uk/
3. FACT-JACIE International Standards for Cellular Therapy Product Collection, Processing and Administration (current edition). http://www.jacie.org/.
4. Human Tissue Act (2004) - http://www.hta.gov.uk/legislationpoliciesandcodesofpractice/legislation/humanti ssueact.cfm
5. EU Directive on Setting Standards of Quality and Safety for the Donation, Procurement, Testing, Processing, Preservation, Storage and distribution of Human Tissues and Cells.

    http://www.ebmt.org/8TransplantGuidelines/tguide8.html.
6. HTA Codes of Practice and Directions. http://www.hta.gov.uk/

3.9   Self Assessment Questions

Multiple Choice Questions

1. What does GMP stand for?
   a) General Medicinal Pharmaceuticals
   b) Good Manufacturing Practice
   c) Good Manufacturing Procedures
   d) Good Medicinal Products
   e) Good Manufacturing Policy

2. GMP covers which of the following practices?
   a) Staff recruitment
   b) Design and use of laboratories
   c) Process validation
   d) Training
   e) Document control

3. Which of the following activities are covered by the EU Tissues and Cell Directive?
   a) Donor selection
   b) Storage
   c) Labelling
   d) Import and export
   e) Donor testing

4. Which of the following are included in the EU Tissues and Cells Directive?
   a) Haematopoietic stem cells
   b) Corneas
   c) Liver
   d) Bone
   e) Skin

Short Answer Questions

1. What key activities are covered by the EU Tissue and Cells Directive? Which cells and tissue are included? Which are excluded?

2. Using the HTA Directions, GMP principles etc what are the key points when storing tissue for therapeutic use?

Assignments

1. Your tissue bank has been asked by a local hospital to bank samples of ovarian tissue intended for implantation into patients. Describe the way in which your tissue bank and the hospital will need to work together to ensure compliance with GMP and the EU Tissues and Cells Directive.

2. Describe the various activities undertaken by your tissue bank or stem cell laboratory which are subject to an external quality assessment scheme. How does your laboratory use data from the scheme to maintain and improve standards?

4 THE COLLECTION, USE AND PROTECTION OF DATA

Data may exist in electronic or physical forms. This includes media such as paper, printouts, fax, databases, tapes, discs, e-mail, microfilm and CDs as well as conversations.

Tissue banks and stem cell laboratories collect and use information and data relating to individuals. As such they are classed as a "data controllers" and have a legal obligation to be registered with the Office of the Data Protection Commissioner. This chapter sets out the main principles and policies governing data handling within tissue banks and stem cell laboratories.

4.1 Freedom of Information Act

The Freedom of Information Act 2000 owes its origins to the European Union principle of transparency - that open government and greater accountability of public bodies secures a higher quality of democracy. The UK Act was fully implemented in January 2005. The UK Act applies to England, Wales and Northern Ireland. The Information Commissioner oversees the implementation and enforcement of the UK Act.

In broad terms, the UK Act sets out an information right i.e. a right of access by the public to all information held by a public authority such as the NHSBT.

The Acts set out two means by which such information held by a public authority may be accessed - via the public authority's publication scheme and via a right to request information. Public authorities must respond to a request for information within 20 working days of receiving it. Information may not necessarily be released if it is subject to an exemption. In other words, the release of such information would not be in the public interest.

Key points for tissue bank and stem cell laboratory staff to bear in mind are:
* Records are open to the public and to the people they are about;
* A record is only of value if its contents are accurate and complete;
* It is a criminal offence for a public authority to alter, damage, erase, destroy or conceal any record they hold once someone has asked for information with the intention of preventing release of the information.

4.2 HTA Directions Regarding Data Protection and Confidentiality

Under the EU Tissues and Cells Directive, the HTA requires that establishments:
* have SOPs to ensure that information provided in confidence is kept confidential;
* ensure data is rendered anonymous before being made available to third parties;
* have SOPs controlling access to confidential data and authorisation to amend data;
* ensure patients and donors are aware of their rights under the Data Protection Act 1988 to access data about themselves;
* records must allow for full traceability. All records including raw data must be kept for a minimum of 10 years. All traceability records must be kept for a minimum of 30 years.

4.3   Confidentiality, Data Protection, Caldicott Principles

All staff should be familiar with their organisational confidentiality and data protection policies and procedures. The NHS places great emphasis on the need for the strictest confidentiality in respect of personal health data. This applies to manual and computer records and conversations about patients' treatments. Everyone working for the NHS is under a legal duty to keep patients' information, held in whatever form, confidential.

The NHS works in line with the eight data protection principles as laid down in the 1998 Data Protection Act (see below).

Patients have a right to know what is happening to their information. Patients can request a copy of personal information held about them under the Data Protection Act 1998 - Subject Access (live patients' information only). Deceased patients' information is also treated as confidential. Disclosure of deceased patients' information must be a matter for individual decision by the clinician. Access is via the Access to Health Records Act 1990 (deceased patients' information only).

4.3.1   Data Protection Principles

The eight data protection principles as laid down in the 1998 Data Protection Act (along with the Caldicott Principles) must be followed at all times. Personal data, in written or electronic form must be:

1. Fairly and lawfully processed;
2. Processed for limited purposes;
3. Adequate, relevant and not excessive for the purpose;
4. Accurate;
5. Kept no longer than necessary;
6. Processed in accordance with the data subject's rights;
7. Secure;
8. Only transferred to countries with adequate data protection systems.

4.3.2   The Caldicott Principles

The Caldicott Principles as laid down by the NHS Executive must also be followed by tissue banking and stem cell laboratory staff. These principles are additional to the Data Protection Act and are intended to regulate access to medical information. Each organisation or Trust will have a "Caldicott Guardian".

Principle 1 - Justify the purpose(s)
Every proposed use or transfer of patient-identifiable information within or from an organisation should be clearly defined and scrutinised, with continuing uses regularly reviewed by an appropriate guardian.

Principle 2 - Don't use patient-identifiable information unless it is absolutely necessary
Patient-identifiable information items should not be used unless there is no alternative.

Principle 3 - Use the minimum necessary patient-identifiable information
Where use of patient-identifiable information is considered to be essential, each individual item of information should be justified with the aim of reducing identifiability.

Principle 4 - Access to patient-identifiable information should be on a strict need to know basis
Only those individuals who need access to patient-identifiable information should have access to it, and they should only have access to the information items that they need to see.

Principle 5 - Everyone should be aware of their responsibilities
Action should be taken to ensure that those handling patient-identifiable information - both clinical and non-clinical staff - are aware of their responsibilities and obligations to respect patient confidentiality.

Principle 6 - Understand and comply with the law
Every use of patient-identifiable information must be lawful. Failure to maintain patient information in a confidential manner can result in disciplinary proceedings being taken against a member of staff.

4.4 The Nature of Personal Data

Data collected, stored and analysed by tissue banks and stem cell laboratories takes several forms as set out below.

Personal data is information about living people which in isolation or in combination with other data which may be available, may lead to the identification of the patient.

Confidential information in the context of healthcare, is information about oneself given on the explicit or implicit understanding that it will not be disclosed to others outside the patient's care, without the patient's consent. Both the law and patients assume that this is the case when personal information is disclosed as part of clinical care.

Sensitive information refers to information about individuals which may have particularly deleterious effects if it is disclosed inappropriately. The Data Protection Act 1998 refers to 'sensitive personal data' as including all information about physical or mental health or condition, or sexual life.

Coded data is not anonymous data. Identities are disguised by the code but the code can be easily decoded by those in control of the data. For example, an 'alphanumeric code' made up of a patient's postcode/initials and date of birth is not anonymous. Informed consent from the participants is required for this situation.

Anonymised data is data which has been coded by others outside the research team, for example from a national database such as the Cancer Registry. Permission for this data to be used in future research should be requested at the time of initial consent to registration or research.

Linked Anonymised data can be decoded by the organisation supplying it to the researchers but not by the researchers themselves. For example a healthcare organisation may need to link perhaps unexpected research data to a particular patient in the interests of their care. Informed consent from the patient is sometimes necessary when using linked anonymous data. The research ethics committee should be consulted.

Unlinked Anonymised data describes the situation where the link between the data and the person to whom it refers has been irreversibly broken. No one could use this data to identify a specific individual. Informed consent is not necessary for research which makes use of unlinked Anonymised data.

4.5 Data Handling within Tissue Banks and Stem Cell Laboratories

The following points should be borne in mind when handling patient-related data.

- Do gain ethical approval for all research using personal and anonymised data;
- Do gain consent from individuals to use their data unless otherwise approved by a research ethics committee;
- Do obtain information from a Caldicott Guardian before undertaking research using existing patient-identifiable data;
- Do treat data as confidential at all times;
- Do anonymise data wherever possible;
- Do password protect and back-up electronic data;
- Do ensure all researchers have full or honorary contracts before allowing access to data. Do ensure data is stored securely for a minimum of 30 years;
- Do not store NHS identifiable information on home computers, laptops, hand held devices etc.;
- Do not store identifiable information on floppy disks or CDs;
- Do not send identifiable information via the internet to an e-mail address that does not end in ".nhs.uk" unless encrypted;
- Do not allow unauthorised persons access to data.

4.6 Further Reading

NHS Confidentiality Code of Practice. Available on line at
http://www.dh.gov.uk/en/Publicationsandstatistics/Publications/PublicationsPolicyAndGuidance/DH_4069253

HTA Codes of Practice on:

- Consent
- Donation of Organs, Tissue and Cells for Transplantation
- Removal Storage and Disposal of Human Organs and Tissue
- Donation of Allogeneic Bone Marrow and Peripheral Blood Stem Cells for transplantation.
http://www.hta.gov.uk/guidance/codes_of_practice.cfm

- For Scotland, the Human Tissue (Scotland) Act 2006 is available at
http://www.opsi.gov.uk/legislation/scotland/acts2006/asp_20060004_en_1

4.7   Self Assessment Questions

Multiple Choice Questions

1. According to the EU Tissues and Cells Directive, records must be kept for a minimum of:
   a) 12 years
   b) 7 years
   c) 25 years
   d) 21 years
   e) 30 years

2. Under which Act can deceased patients' information be disclosed?
   a) Data Protection Act 1998
   b) Freedom of Information Act 2000
   c) Access to Health Records Act 1990
   d) Caldicott Principles Act 1998
   e) Human Tissue Act 2004

3. Which of the following do not require consent from the living?
   a) Obtaining scientific or medical information which may be relevant to any other person, now or in the future;
   b) Research in connection with disorders, or the functioning of the human body;
   c) Public display
   d) Transplantation
   e) Clinical audit

4. Which of the following people can lawfully give consent?
   a) A child under 18 years old
   b) Deceased person's nominated representative
   c) Spouse or partner
   d) Parent or child
   e) All of the above

Short Answer Questions

1. List the eight principles set out in the Data Protection Act

2. What is meant by 'scheduled purposes' under the Human Tissue Act.

Assignments

1. Your tissue bank or stem cell laboratory has decided to procure an IT system to help improve the traceability of products and processes. The system will hold confidential data on patients and donors. Prepare an outline specification to ensure IT system is designed to protect confidentiality of stored data.

2. Your tissue bank or stem cell laboratory has donor tissue in cryogenic storage which was originally donated for therapeutic use only. This tissue is now past its expiry data and staff at a local university department would like to use some of it for research. The data generated might have medical implications for the donors concerned. Prepare an outline submission for your local ethics committee describing how you would intend to anonymise the data and any proposals you may have regarding donor consent for the study.

5 DONOR SCREENING AND TESTING

5.1 Infectious Agents

5.1.1 Background

Stem cell and tissue products like all blood products are capable of transmitting infectious agents to the recipient. Viruses, bacteria, prions and protozoa have all been demonstrated to be transmitted by transfusion of blood or blood products. For an agent to be transmitted by transfusion it needs to give rise to asymptomatic infection, be present in the blood stream, be transmitted parenterally and be able to survive during storage.

5.1.2 Viruses

There are several groups of viruses known to be transmitted by transfusion but not all undergo mandatory testing. Hepatitis viruses are a diverse group that includes hepadenoviruses, flaviviruses and picornaviruses. Hepatitis B virus is a DNA virus and a member of the hepadenovirus family. These types of virus are characterised by the production of large amounts of surface proteins together with the infectious particles (DNA genome encapsulated in core protein and surrounded by an envelope of surface proteins). Following parental transmission to the recipient there may be an acute infection where an immune response is mounted or a chronic infection with persistence of viral replication.

Hepatitis C virus is an enveloped RNA virus within the flavivirus family. Infection can be acute followed by resolution or chronic and persistent. HCV RNA and HCV antigen can be detected in infected individuals. There are several genotypes that appear to be geographically associated and that also show some variation in the course and severity of infection.

Human Immunodeficiency Virus is a retrovirus that primarily infects lymphocytes in particular CD4 T cells. After infecting the lymphocytes the virus integrates into the cell DNA and then replicates. Following the initial infection most people recover after a few weeks then seroconvert and appear to remain asymptomatic although there may be an underlying chronic infection. There then can be a gradual decline in numbers of CD4 T cells so that the infected individual eventually becomes susceptible to opportunistic infections leading to acquired immune deficiency syndrome. There have been a number of types and subtypes of HIV identified the major division being into types I and II.

Human T cell leukaemia virus-I was the first human retrovirus identified. It is an oncogenic virus causing adult T-cell leukaemia and lymphoma and tropical spastic paraparesis. A second virus HTLV-II has been identified associated with specific groups of individuals such as drug users but no specific disease process has yet been associated with it. Most infections with HTLV are asymptomatic although disease can occur at anytime after infection. Like HIV it is thought HTLV is cell associated again infecting CD4 positive lymphocytes and is transmitted in these cells. Seroconversion occurs between 30 and 90 days following infection and prior to this viral RNA can be found in lymphocytes. Once seroconversion has occurred the antibodies generally persist for life.

5.1.3 Bacteria and fungi

Although bacterial contamination of blood products is uncommon post-transfusion bacterial sepsis has a high mortality rate. Bacterial contamination in blood and stem cells may be derived endogenously (e.g. from bacteria circulating in the donor's blood such as *Treponema pallidum* and *Yersinia enterocolitica)* or exogenously (e.g. from bacteria entering the product during collection or processing). The latter may include Pseudomonas and *Staphylococcus* organisms. Bacterial and fungal contamination is however more common in tissue, where the tissue is retrieved in post mortem room and from donors who have died traumatically. Whereas blood and stem cells can be retrieved under near sterile conditions, removal of bone and heart valves require cutting through the donor's skin which can lead to increased contamination. As skin and corneas are external tissues they will have an associated flora of bacteria and fungi   at all times

5.1.4 Treponema pallidum

These spirochaetes are the causative agent of syphilis. Syphilis can lead to several stages following infection and although the primary site of infection can heal there may be continuing infection in the regional lymph glands, which remains unless treated correctly. The treponemes are released into the blood as part of their life cycle but are sensitive to heat being destroyed at 4 degrees C. The spirochaetes can only be found in the blood for short periods of time; identification of infected individuals relies on serology.

5.1.5 Prions

Creutzfeldt-Jakob disease (CJD) is a rare and ultimately fatal progressive degenerative brain disease. It is one of a group of diseases called Transmissible Spongiform Encephalopathies (TSEs) that affect humans and animals. TSEs are thought to be caused by the build up in the brain of an abnormal form of the naturally occurring 'prion' protein.

CJD was initially described in its classical, or sporadic form, in 1920. A new variant known as variant CJD (vCJD) was first identified in 1996. Variant CJD is strongly linked to exposure, probably through food, to a TSE of cattle called Bovine Spongiform Encephalopathy (BSE). Although there have been no reported cases of vCJD having been transmitted as a result of surgical procedures, the possibility cannot be ruled out. Precautionary measures have been taken to reduce such a risk by improving the standards of decontamination services for surgical instruments.

There have been several cases of vCJD infection associated with blood transfusion with some recipients developing symptoms of vCJD. The possibility that vCJD can be transmitted through blood raises concern about the possible infectivity of blood components and plasma products.

5.2   Testing

The UK Blood Services collect and test blood donations for five mandated infectious diseases (HIV, HBV, HCV, HTLV and syphilis), and other discretionary tests may be applied (e.g., malaria, Chagas). The standard approach aims for a system which maximises sensitivity in the first (initial), highly automated high-throughput testing step and specificity in the final (confirmatory) low-through-put specialised testing step. Standard practice is to undertake a repeat test (in duplicate) on any sample which is reactive in the initial screen.

Blood and (living) tissue donors (including stem cell donors) consent to their blood being tested. They also consent to knowing the results of tests performed on their donations that may affect their health. In the case of deceased donors of tissues, most tissue banks inform relatives if results are deemed relevant to their own health.

5.2.1 Regulatory Aspects

All donors of bone marrow or peripheral blood stem cells must be tested for mandated infectious diseases within a 30 day period prior to harvest. For donors of tissues and cells, testing must include Hepatitis B core. Results must be available before conditioning therapy in the stem cell recipient is initiated and any tissues are implanted

Living tissue donors must be tested within 7 days of surgery for mandated infectious diseases. The blood sample can be tested using PCR; if is not available then the donor must have a follow up blood sample taken 180 days post surgery.

Deceased donors must have a blood sample taken within 24 hours of death. The blood sample must be obtained away from any intravenous sites to ensure that there is no haemodilution. A haemodilution calculation is performed to ensure that the blood sample is representative of the serological status of the donor. If the patient has received blood, plasma or platelet infusion within 7 days of their death, a pretransfusion blood sample is preferable. If available, a blood sample taken in the 24 hours before death is preferable to a post mortem one.

5.2.2 Testing for Viruses

All microbiological tests must be highly sensitive with a high degree of specificity to avoid false positives. Furthermore, all positive tests require further confirmatory testing to ensure a true positive result. Most viral serology tests are enzyme immunoassay based. These assays have been developed to improve sensitivity in both antigen presentation e.g. bead technology and detection with more sensitive antibodies aimed at both the IgG and IgM components of the immune response. Testing for Hepatitis B does not involve detection of antibody but that of the surface antigen released into the blood of the individual. The aim of developing the modern assay is to reduce the so-called window period. This is the time during which the patient may be infectious and asymptomatic without the presence of antibodies or viral antigen for detection. Nucleic Acid Amplification Technology (NAT testing) is now implemented to detect viral DNA or RNA. This technology has the theoretical potential of identifying viral infection at an earlier stage. Enzyme assays for HCV have a window phase of around 70 days; this can be reduced to below 11 days by NAT testing. Most systems used are automated and a typical system uses the Qiagen BioRobot 9604 for extraction and the COBAS Ampliscreen HCV assay for amplification and detection. The system uses an internal control - an *in vitro* RNA transcript with the same primer binding sites as the HCV sequence. Biotinylated primers are used for the detection of the amplified products. Using this system a 95% assay sensitivity for HCV RNA of 12IU/ml has been achieved.

5.2.3 Testing for Cytomegalovirus

Most humans are exposed to cytomegalovirus in their lifetime, but typically only individuals with weakened immune systems (i.e. post chemotherapy or BMT) become ill. The majority of adults have antibodies (an indication of previous infection) to CMV by age 40. Serious CMV infections can include pneumonia, gastroenteritis, retinitis and encephalitis. CMV-negative stem cell donors (and blood donors) may be donors of choice for CMV-negative recipients.

Testing for CMV is based on antibody detection in donor plasma or serum.

5.2.4 Testing for Bacteria in Stem Cell Products

Bacterial contamination of the stem cell product may arise because of donor bacteraemia, contamination during the collection, contamination of the collection pack and contamination during the processing. It is during collection that the majority of contamination events arise often related to normal skin flora. As stem cell products are normally frozen or transfused relatively quickly after collection the levels of bacteria in most cases are low and can be controlled by antibiotics once detected. Therefore, a good method of detection is required. A variety of testing methods can be used to detect bacterial contamination of stem cell products but the most sensitive and until now probably the best suited is Bactalert™, a fully automated blood culture system. The system works by firstly, inoculating a Bactalert bottle with a sample from the stem cell product; any micro-organisms will then multiply and generate CO_2. As CO_2 levels increase a sensor in the bottle turns yellow; the automated reader can detect this colour change. Both aerobic and anaerobic cultures are set up and these are incubated for a minimum of seven days for automated reading and 14 days for visual detection to allow for the detection of fungal contamination.

5.2.5 Testing for Bacteria in Tissue Products

The type and length of bacterial tests depends on the tissue.

Corneas are used the soonest after procurement and therefore have an abbreviated test. Being a surface graft and not exposed to blood stream corneas are not as critical if low levels of bacteria and fungi are present. For corneas being stored at +4°C sample of sclera are taken and reports are produced at 24 and 48 hours with final report at 1 week. Corneas stored at +4°C will be issued on a no-growth report at 24 hours as corneas at this temperature have a 7 day expiry. Corneas in organ culture at 34°C have the media tested at 7 days and after transfer into dextran medium.

For bone, samples of excised tissue are taken and cultured both aerobically and anaerobically on Horse Blood Agar and on Sabouraud Agar for 7 days. The bone is rejected if there is confluent growth but donations with no growth, scanty growth or moderate growth are reported as pass. Bone is gamma irradiated after the test has taken place so this will act as the sterilisation phase.

For skin, samples are placed in Tryptone Soya Broth and Thioglycollate broths at both pre and post antibiotic treatment stages. The presence of non pathogenic organisms in either pre or post decontamination sampling does not contraindicate transplantation and will be reported as pass. If specific pathogenic organisms are identified in the pre sample the tissue is reported as "suitable for irradiation" If specific pathogenic organisms are identified in the post samples then the tissue is reported as fail. The specific pathogenic organisms include Pseudomonas aeruginosa, Staphylococcus aureus, Clostridium species, Mycobacterium tuberculi, pyogenic streptococci and fungi.

For heart valves, the transport medium and samples post antibiotic treatment and at time of cryopreservation are tested. The samples of the tissue are placed in glucose broth, Fashelious anaerobic broth and Sabourauds broth and the broths and the transport medium are plated out on to blood agar, aerobic and anaerobic, or Sabourauds plates after 6 days. The presence of pathogenic organisms, similar to those listed above in the transport medium leads to discard of the tissue. Bacterial or fungal growth after antibiotic treatment or at time of freezing also leads to discard. Most heart valve banks also perform a specific test for mycobacteria and any evidence of M. tuberculi leads also to discard.

5.2.6   Testing for Prions

Tests for vCJD in the blood of asymptomatic individuals are being developed. Tests that can be applied to tissues (but not to blood) have already been used in anonymised epidemiological studies.

It is reasonable to assume that a test for vCJD will be mandated by the Department of Health once a test becomes feasible (even if the true effectiveness of the test is unknown). This 'precautionary approach' reflects legal precedents set following reviews of HIV and HCV testing of blood donations.

NHSBT have been testing deceased tissue donors for vCJD using tonsil tissue as an analyte. There are operational restrictions with using tonsillar tissue for testing (for example, opening the donor's mouth post-mortem) which have led to the investigation into changing the analyte. An operational feasibility study is being planned into the testing of spleen and ocular tissue from deceased tissue donors for vCJD.

5.3   Suggested Reading

1. *Introduction to Modern Virology.* Dimmock NJ, Easton AJ, Leppard KN (eds).
2. *Practical Hematopoietic Stem Cell Transplantation.* Cant AJ, Galloway A, Jackson G (eds). Pages 55 to 80
3. Health Protection Agency information on vCJD and prion testing. http://www.hpa.org.uk/infections/topics_az/cjd/blood_products.htm
4. Guidelines for the Blood Transfusion Services in the UK (7th edition). Chapters 10 (Microbiology Tests for Donors and Donations), 22 (Tissue Banking) and 24 (Haemopoietic Stem Cells). http://www.transfusionguidelines.org.uk/
5. Department of Health, Advisory Committee on the Microbiological Safety of Blood and Tissues for Transplantation. Guidance on the Microbiological Safety of Human Organs, Tissues and Cells used in Transplantation (August 2000). http://www.dh.gov.uk/prod_consum_dh/groups/dh_digitalassets/@dh/@en/docume nts/digitalasset/dh_4079053.pdf

5.4   Self Assessment Questions

Multiple Choice Questions

1. What does NAT stand for?
    a) National Acceptance Testing
    b) Nucleic Acid Amplification Technology
    c) Nucleic Acid Testing
    d) Nucleic Antibody Test
    e) Nucleic Absorbance Test

2. When must a blood sample for mandatory microbiology testing be taken from a stem cell donor?
    a) Within 7 days of donation
    b) Up to 1 month after donation
    c) At the time of donation
    d) Within 30 days before donation
    e) Six months after donation

3. Which of the following is not a mandatory test for stem cells / tissues?
    a) vCJD
    b) HIV
    c) HTLV
    d) Hepatitis B
    e) Hepatitis C

4. Which of the following statements is false?
    a) Hepatitis C virus is an enveloped RNA virus from the flavivirus family.
    b) NAT testing reduces the window period for seroconversion.
    c) Tissue and cell donors must be tested for Hepatitis B core antigen.
    d) CMV testing is mandatory.
    e) Creutzfeldt-Jakob disease is one of a group of diseases called Transmissible Spongiform Encephalopathy.

Short Answer Questions

1. Why is NAT testing important?
2. What is haemodilution and why must this be considered with respect to deceased tissue donors?

Assignments

1. Why is Nucleic Acid Amplification testing important? What steps need to be taken if a sample tests positive upon initial screen?

2. Compare the main sources of bacterial contamination for stem cell and tissue products?

6 ASEPTIC TECHNIQUE, STERILISATION, IRRADIATION, DISINFECTION AND QUALITY CONTROL FOR TISSUES

6.1 Background

It is good practice, where practical, to sterilise or disinfect tissue grafts before they are implanted. Grafts taken from living donors under operating theatre conditions that are not manipulated before re-implantation are not sterilised or disinfected and therefore must be donated aseptically. The application of sterilisation or disinfection can eliminate or greatly reduce the potential for transmission of disease from the graft to the recipient. This can arise from the donor themselves (for example, septicaemia or blood-borne viruses) or contamination of the graft with environmental micro-organisms during retrieval or subsequent processing procedures. It is important to be aware that even after serology testing of donors, and bacteriological and mycological assessment of tissues, there remains a small but significant risk that transmissible diseases can be present in the tissue. Serological testing may not detect recent 'window period' infections, and can also only be used to test for diseases that are known and for which a valid test exists. Bacteriology/mycology testing of grafts is by its nature a sampling process and may not detect low level contamination.

6.2 Definitions

Aseptic	Absence of germs, infections and septic material, is directed toward cleanliness and the elimination of infectious agents.
Aseptic Technique	The practice that restricts micro-organisms in the environment, on equipment and supplies, and prevents normal body flora from contaminating the surgical field.
Surgical Conscience	Concept that allows no compromise in principles of aseptic technique. Anything less could increase the potential risk of infection. Applies to all members of the team, observed or not.

6.3 Eight Principles of Aseptic Technique

1   All items used within a sterile field must be sterile;
2   A sterile barrier that has been permeated/damaged must be considered contaminated;
3   The edges of a sterile wrapper or container are considered unsterile after the package is open;
4   Gowns are considered sterile in front, from chest to level of the sterile field, and the sleeves are sterile from 2 inches above the elbows to the cuff;

(Scrubbed personnel should pass each other either back to back or front to front)

5   Tables are sterile at table level only;
6   Sterile persons and items only touch sterile areas. Unsterile persons and items touch only unsterile areas;
7   Movement within or around a sterile field must not contaminate the field;
8   All items and areas of doubtful sterility are considered contaminated.

6.4   Aseptic Procedure

Aseptic procedures are used where it is important to minimise risks of microbiological contamination and of particulate and pyrogen contamination. This can be achieved in an environment designed to remove the risk of contamination and the design will depend on the process to be carried out. 'Clean areas' are classified according to the required characteristics of the environment as follows (GMP classifications):

- Grade A: for high risk operations, e.g. open ampoules and vials, making aseptic connections, open processing of tissues. Normally such conditions are provided by a class II microbiological safety cabinet.
- Grade B: for aseptic preparation and filling this provides the background environment for a Grade A zone.
- Grade C&D: clean areas for carrying out less critical stages in the manufacture of sterile products.

The restrictions for airborne particulate matter for each of these grades can be found in the Rules and Guidance for Pharmaceutical Manufacturers and Distributors (Orange Guide (8) in addition to a more comprehensive guide to cleanroom requirements.

Most processing operations involved in tissue banks and stem cell laboratories are classified as 'open' and therefore must be carried out in a Grade A environment, with a validated background.

High levels of personal hygiene and cleanliness are essential when carrying out an aseptic procedure. Each laboratory will have written procedures describing procedures associated with aseptic procedure including a description of clothing required for each grade of work area.

6.5   Sterilisation, Disinfection and Decontamination

The term 'decontamination', which can be defined as rendering a material safe by the removal of infectious pathogenic agents, encompasses both sterilisation and disinfection. Sterilisation is an easier term to define, simply meaning the total destruction or elimination of all micro-organisms, whilst disinfection is more difficult to define precisely. In the context of tissue grafts, it generally refers to the destruction or elimination of pathogenic micro-organisms.

6.6   Sterilisation and Disinfection Methodologies

There are a number of different techniques available for the decontamination of tissue grafts. It should be noted that a given technique can be either a sterilisation or a disinfection protocol, depending on the conditions under which it is applied; for example, gamma irradiation can be a disinfection protocol when applied at low dosages, but a sterilisation protocol at higher dosages. The choice of which decontamination protocol is appropriate for each type of tissue graft is informed by the efficacy of the protocol, and by the deleterious effects it has on the biological and/or biomechanical properties of the graft. Generally speaking, the more effective a protocol is, the more damaging it is to the tissue.

The choice of protocol should therefore be based on an informed risk-benefit analysis that takes into account:

- The probability of a tissue being contaminated - based on the anatomical location of the tissue, the location at which the retrieval takes place and the post mortem time at which it takes place.
- The potential level (bioburden) of contamination on the tissue
- The potential pathogenicity of any contamination
- The deleterious effects of the decontamination process on the tissue properties; the degree of these effects, and how vital the property in question is to clinical performance of the graft.

6.6.1　Chemical decontamination

Chemical decontamination involves the application of chemicals, usually in a gaseous or liquid form, to the tissue. The mode of action is generally the destruction of protein and/or DNA molecules.

A number of different chemicals are used, or have been used in the past to decontaminate tissues. Chemical decontamination treatments range from surface disinfection procedures, such as alcohol wiping, to full sterilisation protocols such as ethylene oxide gas sterilisation. The most commonly used chemical sterilant is gaseous ethylene oxide.

6.6.2　Alcohols

Alcohol solutions, principally ethanol in a 70% aqueous solution, are used both as a surface disinfectant and as a soaking solution. They have multiple modes of action, some of which are best achieved by permitting the alcohol solution to evaporate from the surface being disinfected. Alcohols are most effective against vegetative micro-organisms, but are much less effective against spores. They are often used as carriers for other decontaminating chemicals, such as chlorhexidine gluconate. Alcohol disinfection may be used to treat the skin of deceased tissue donors prior to retrieval of tissues, as a surface swab prior to dissection of heart valves, and as a soak for the treatment of tendon allografts. The advantages of alcohols as disinfectants are that they are relatively mild, and have few deleterious effects on tissue properties. They are also much less toxic than other chemical decontaminants so retention of residuals and staff safety are not major concerns. This is counterbalanced however by the relative weakness and limited range of their antimicrobial activity.

6.6.3　Peroxygen Compounds

Peroxygen compounds, principally hydrogen peroxide and peracetic acid, are popular chemical decontaminants for tissues. They are used either as liquid soaking solutions, or as gas plasmas. When in contact with organic tissue (or certain metal ions) the compounds degrade, releasing reactive oxygen species ('free radicals') which exert killing effects. They have a wide range of activity, being effective versus vegetative micro-organisms, spores and viruses. They are generally supplied as high concentration, stabilised solutions, which are diluted prior to use, either with water or buffered saline. Peracetic acid is more stable than hydrogen peroxide, and has been used extensively for the treatment of musculoskeletal allografts, principally in Germany. A particular preparation of 1% v/v peracetic acid in aqueous ethanol solution has been validated as a sterilisation protocol. In the UK, NHSBT has investigated the application of lower concentration peracetic acid treatment for the decontamination of skin and tendon allografts.

Whilst the treatments performed well in development studies and were shown not to damage the tissues, in routine clinical application their efficacy was inconsistent. NHSBT does however incorporate a wash in 3% hydrogen peroxide into its bone processing protocol, which has been shown to significantly deplete bioburden. The advantages of peroxygen compounds are their efficacy and wide range of action, and the fact that they degrade into non-toxic chemicals after application; hydrogen peroxide degrades to water and oxygen, and peracetic acid to acetic acid and oxygen. There are thus no concerns regarding residuals remaining in the tissue, or staff safety in their application. Their limitations arise from their damaging effects to tissue structure. These effects depend on the tissue in question; for hard tissues, they are less pronounced, but their use in stress bearing soft tissues, such as tendons or cardiovascular grafts is not advisable without extensive validation.

6.6.4 Chlorine Compounds

Chlorine gas or chlorine compounds are commonly used chemical disinfectants. They are not widely used in the treatment of tissues due to their deleterious effects on tissue properties. However hypochlorite compounds, such as sodium hypochlorite are of interest due to their demonstrated anti-prion properties. The primary mode of action of chlorine, and chlorine based compounds is thought to be their dissolution in aqueous solution to form hypochlorous acid. The high concentrations (>20,000ppm) of hypochlorite required to inactivate prions renders this treatment unsuitable for tissue grafts; soft tissue grafts are partially dissolved by this treatment, and hard grafts are demineralised. It has been used in lower concentrations in the treatment of bone grafts, for its antimicrobial and bleaching effects, and also as a surface decontaminant for skin allografts, but is not widely used for the treatment of tissue grafts.

6.6.5 Glutaraldehyde

Glutaraldehyde is a well characterised chemical decontaminant. It acts by crosslinking intracellular and extracellular proteins, and is effective versus all classes of micro-organisms. When applied to tissues, it crosslinks extracellular matrix proteins which alters the mechanical and biological properties of the tissue. This can be advantageous if the crosslinking strengthens the tissue and makes it more resistant to degradation, but also has adverse effects as tissue thus treated is prone to calcify *in vivo*. Glutaraldehyde is also a carcinogen, which can leach out of an implanted graft over time. In tissue banking, glutaraldehyde has been used historically to treat dura mater and other membrane type grafts, but is rarely if at all used today, owing to concerns regarding toxic residuals and *in vivo* calcification. It is used commercially for the preparation of xenogeneic heart valve grafts, derived from porcine tissue. In this situation, its excellent antimicrobial properties justify the use of xenogeneic tissue, and the crosslinking of the tissue lengthens the lifespan of the graft. However, *in vivo* calcification is a drawback with these grafts.

6.6.6 Ethylene Oxide

Ethylene oxide is a toxic alkylating agent that is widely used to sterilize heat labile medical equipment. It has a broad range of activity, and is effective versus all classes of micro-organisms. It is predominantly used as a gas, either at 37 or 55°C, and therefore one of its restrictions when applied to tissues is that the tissue must be dry before exposure. The presence of fluids in the tissue hinder gas penetration, and in the case of ethylene oxide also result in the formation of toxic by-products such as ethylene chlorohydrin and ethylene glycol that can persist in the tissue. It is therefore used to sterilize lyophilised tissues, predominantly bone allografts although it has been used in the past to treat other freeze dried allografts, such as tendon and skin. Its efficacy, combined with the availability of commercial sterilizers and the fact that it has no deleterious effects on the mechanical properties of the tissue made it a popular choice for these grafts. As a gaseous sterilant, it is also easier to remove from tissues after use by aeration at high ambient temperature.

Until recently, this was the sterilant of choice for processed bone allografts as a reliable, broad spectrum sterilant that did not damage the tissue structural properties, it was ideal for this purpose. The only significant safety concern was the potential retention of residual amounts of ethylene oxide or its by-products in the tissue after sterilisation, and it was necessary to periodically validate the sterilisation protocol to ensure that these residuals were below a maximum safe level. However, recent advice from the Department of Health, to the effect that there was no effective safe level of residual ethylene oxide, and that it should only be used where there was no other alternative, has led to its replacement with gamma irradiation for sterilization of bone grafts. Currently, ethylene oxide sterilization is only permitted for weight bearing allografts.

6.6.7   Antibiotic Decontamination

Antibiotic decontamination involves soaking tissues in a solution of antibiotics, usually prepared in a buffered, physiological solution. This is a relatively weak disinfection process, which is only used in the treatment of tissues where cell viability is required, as it is the only decontamination process that will selectively target micro-organisms over cells.

The antibiotic solution is prepared at the point of use, or in some cases prepared earlier and frozen until required. It generally comprises a range of different antibiotics, including at least one anti-fungal compound, selected to have as wide a range of activity as possible against micro-organisms. The antibiotics are dissolved in a physiological, buffered solution, selected so as to minimise cell damage due to changes in osmotic pressure or pH. The tissue grafts are immersed in the antibiotic solution, with or without agitation, for a set period of time. Incubation times of between 12 and 24 hours are most common. The temperature at which the incubation is performed varies, usually temperatures of *circa* 4°C, room temperature or 37°C are selected. Higher incubation temperatures are usually associated with shorter incubation times; antibiotic cocktails are usually more effective at higher temperatures, but this can result in a reduction of tissue viability due to increased autodegradation, and antibiotic toxicity. It is important to test the bacteriological status of the tissue both before and after disinfection, as antibiotic residuals in the tissue can compromise post-disinfection results

Antibiotic disinfection is the method of choice for disinfecting grafts where cell viability is thought to be important for optimal graft performance, and was initially developed to treat cardiovascular allografts. It is also used to treat skin and meniscal grafts where cell viability is desirable. However, it has the following limitations:

- It is a relatively weak disinfection process; using standard bacteriological and mycological acceptance criteria, the disinfection processes is unsuccessful for between a quarter and a third of grafts.
- It is established that antibiotic residues bind to the graft during disinfection; this can compromise post-process microbiological assessments, and raises potential patient safety issues where a recipient has an allergic response to any of the antibiotics in the cocktail
- Even though the disinfection process is designed to maintain cell viability, the antibiotic cocktails used are toxic to cells and the severity of the disinfection (in terms of temperature and incubation time) must be minimised to reduce these effects
- Antibiotic solutions have no anti-viral activities

     42

6.6.8 Gamma Irradiation

Gamma irradiation is a physical decontamination method in which the material to be sterilised is exposed to high energy gamma rays from a decaying radioactive source (usually cobalt[60]). Gamma irradiation has two principle modes of action. The primary effect is when gamma rays (high energy photons) directly impact with molecules. When this occurs, covalent bonds within the molecules can be broken apart, inactivating biological molecules. This mode of action is particularly effective against nucleic acid molecules and proteins which are comparatively large and thus more likely to be hit by the gamma rays. The secondary effect occurs when a gamma ray impacts with a water molecule. This generates short lived but highly destructive reactive oxygen species (free radicals) which also damage molecules and promote protein cross linking.

Gamma irradiation is also used to sterilise a wide variety of medical consumables, such as bandages and syringes. It is generally a service offered by third party companies as it requires a separate specialist plant. In these plants, the radioactive source is contained within a thick concrete core, which is connected to an adjoining warehouse via a conveyor belt. Items to be sterilised are loaded onto the conveyor belt, which runs into the core and around the source so that all surfaces are equally exposed to the core. The conveyor belt then returns the sterilised items to the warehouse. The radiation dose received by the items is controlled by the speed of the conveyor belt, i.e. when it runs slowly, the items remain in the core for longer and receive a greater radiation dose.

Gamma irradiation has been used to sterilise a number of different tissue grafts. It is primarily used to treat musculoskeletal grafts, where it has the advantage of being able to easily penetrate to the centre of the graft, even through thick cortical bone. It is also used to treat tendon allografts, and occasionally other types of graft. Gamma irradiation has recently been introduced to treat contaminated skin grafts, although in this case it was necessary to treat the skin with a radioprotective chemical (glycerol) to ameliorate the secondary effects of irradiation. The advantages of its application are that unlike chemical sterilants it does not leave any residual components in the tissue (although the irradiation process can generate toxic compounds in tissue, for example the generation of lipid peroxides in bone marrow). The effects of irradiation on connective tissue proteins is complex; the primary effects cause scission of chemical bonds and weakening of the protein, whereas the secondary effects cause the proteins to cross link, making the matrix stiffer.

Irradiation leads to a dose dependent reduction in the mechanical strength of structural tissue grafts. For this reason, many surgeons will not use irradiated grafts because of the risk of early mechanical failure. Efforts have been made to address these concerns - one approach has been to reduce the dose of irradiation applied to grafts, justified by assessing the bioburden present before irradiation. Another has been to impregnate the tissue with a cocktail of radioprotective chemicals prior to irradiation, to ameliorate the secondary effects. It is also less effective against certain classes of micro-organisms, in particular bacterial spores and viruses. Where contamination with these organisms is suspected, higher dosages need to be applied.

6.6.9 Heat

Heat, either alone or in combination with steam and pressure can be used to sterilise or disinfect. The most common form of heat sterilisation, autoclaving, can not be used to sterilise tissues as it is too destructive to the mechanical and biological properties of tissue. It is however very useful for the sterilisation of single use and re-useable instruments. Milder forms of heat disinfection (pasteurisation) can be applied to tissues however.

Autoclaving, or steam sterilisation, requires exposure of an item to steam at high pressure and temperature. By containing the items to be sterilised in a sealed pressure vessel and increasing the heat in the presence of water, superheated steam is created which penetrates the items quickly and kills micro-organisms. A pressure of 15psi generates steam at a temperature of 121°C is effective against all classes of micro-organisms. Although some classes, such as bacterial spores are more resistant.

Pasteurisation is a more gentle heat treatment, requiring heating of an item to a temperature of generally between 50 and 80°C for a defined period of time. The treatment time varies in accordance with the temperature, with higher temperatures requiring a shorter treatment time. To ensure even temperature distribution and to guard against accidental overheating, the item is usually immersed in fluid prior to treatment. Pasteurisation is not a sterilisation technique, but is effective against vegetative bacteria, fungi and viruses. Bacterial and fungal spores are resistant to pasteurisation.

Autoclaving is not considered a viable process for tissues, due to its immensely destructive effects on both biological and mechanical properties. It has been used historically in some situations to treat bone allografts that are not intended to have a weight or stress bearing properties, but not for some time. It used to be common practice to incorporate a pasteurisation step (55-60°C, 3-4 hours) at the beginning of bone processing protocols, to reduce initial bioburden prior to processing and to protect processing staff from any viral contaminants in the tissue. However, improvements in the asepsis of tissue retrieval, and of donor selection and screening protocols led to this process being removed. A commercial pasteurisation system was also developed and marketed by a German company in the 1990s, aimed at pasteurising femoral heads by heating to 80°C for 30 minutes. This was developed to allow hospital based bone banks without processing facilities to pasteurise their own grafts. However, pasteurisation, even at lower temperatures has deleterious effects on soft tissues and is only applicable to bone grafts, where the connective tissue proteins are afforded some protection by the mineralised matrix.

6.7   Validation and Checking/Quality Control

Decontamination is a critical process, and as such must be validated to ensure that it is achieving the claimed result. In the case of disinfection processes, such as antibiotic disinfection, complete microbial killing can not be guaranteed in every case. In these situations, the microbiological status of the tissue must be assessed by sampling each batch and culturing the samples for bacterial and fungal growth, usually both before and after disinfection. Microbiological acceptance criteria for tissues treated in this way need to be developed, in order to relate the potential risk of transmitting pathogenic micro-organisms to the recipient to the benefits of the graft.

Where a sterilisation process is applied, it is expected that all micro-organisms will be killed. This assertion must be supported by validation proving that the process is capable of inactivating a defined bioburden. This bioburden must be based on the normal bioburden found on the graft in question (which can only be determined by testing a large number of samples) and also include an overkill factor (Sterility Assurance Level, or SAL) of 10^{-6}. This means that the sterilisation process must kill the entire existing bioburden, plus achieve an additional six $\log^{10}$ reductions in microbe number as a safety margin. A $\log^{10}$ reduction is the reduction of the number of microbes by 90%; therefore a six log reduction equates to a 99.9999% reduction. When this is applied after elimination of the existing bioburden, it reduces the chances that a graft could be contaminated to one in one million.

The dose of sterilisation required to achieve this is called the D^{10} value. For example, if bioburden studies tell us that the most resistant micro-organism associated with a graft is a bacterial spore, present at a maximum level of 10,000 organisms per graft, then the sterilisation dosage must be 10 times the D^{10} value. Obviously, we must also know the D^{10} value for the organism with respect to the particular sterilisation treatment. In the example above, if the tissue is to be irradiated and we know the D^{10} value for that organism to be 2 kGy, a minimum dosage of 20kGy would need to be applied.

Where a sterilisation process is well validated and well controlled, it is not necessary to physically test samples of the tissue to confirm sterility. If it can be confirmed that the process has been performed according to its validated specification, it can be assumed that the tissue is sterile. This is called parametric release, and is commonly applied to irradiation sterilisation and autoclaving where the physical parameters of the process can be accurately recorded. This process can only be applied to grafts that are terminally sterilised in their final packaging.

6.8   Water Measurement (Available Water)

This test is used for the measurement of water activity within freeze dried tissue. The water content of a substance (residual moisture) is usually measured gravimetrically by drying the substance until no further weight loss is achieved and expressing the residual weight as a percentage of the original substance weight. In contrast to water content, water activity (Aw) is defined as a measurement of the energy status of the water in a system and indicates how tightly the water is bound within that system. It is equal to the equilibrium relative humidity (ERH) and a high Aw (>0.8 indicates a 'wet' system and a low Aw (<0.7) indicates a 'dry' system. This can be used to predict product safety and stability with respect to microbial growth, biochemical reaction rates and physical properties. Determination and control of water activity, rather than water content, is very important as low water activity prevents microbial growth (Figure 1). A water activity of about 0.6Aw denotes a cessation of microbial growth although this figure is somewhat dependent on the solutes present: For example glycerol efficiently lowers water activity but may still allow microbial growth and consequently a lower water activity may be required. A water activity of 0.3Aw is optimal for minimising lipid oxidation, enzyme activity and hydrolytic reactions. The limit of water activity for freeze dried bone is 0.5 Aw.

Figure 1. Effect of Water Content on Biological Activity

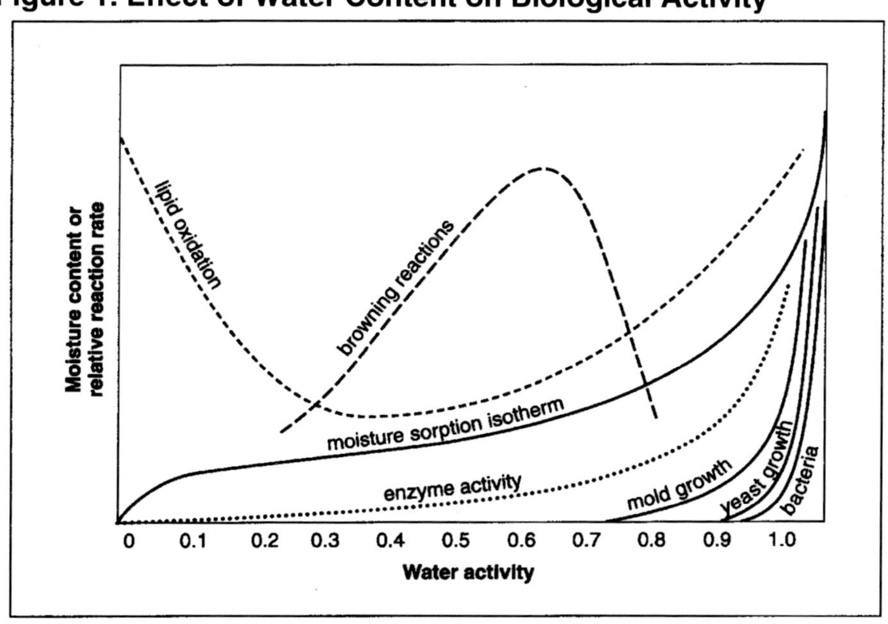

Fig 1.   Relationship between water activity and moisture content.
(adapted from Labuza *et al*; Adv.Exp.Med Biol(1977):<u>86b</u>:379-418)

6.8.1 Measurement of Water Activity

The Pawkit has been designed to be a simple, rapid and portable system for measurement of water activity. Briefly, a tissue sample is placed in a sample cup which is sealed inside a chamber (Figures 2 and 3). Water activity is measured by equilibrating the liquid phase water in the sample with the vapour phase water in the headspace and then measuring the relative humidity of the headspace. As the relative humidity of the chamber changes, the electrical conductance of a dielectric sensor in the chamber changes, from which the relative humidity can be computed. When the water activity (Aw) of the sample and the relative humidity of the air are in equilibrium the measurement of the headspace humidity gives the water activity of the sample.

Figure 2. Pawkit Meter for Determination of Water Activity

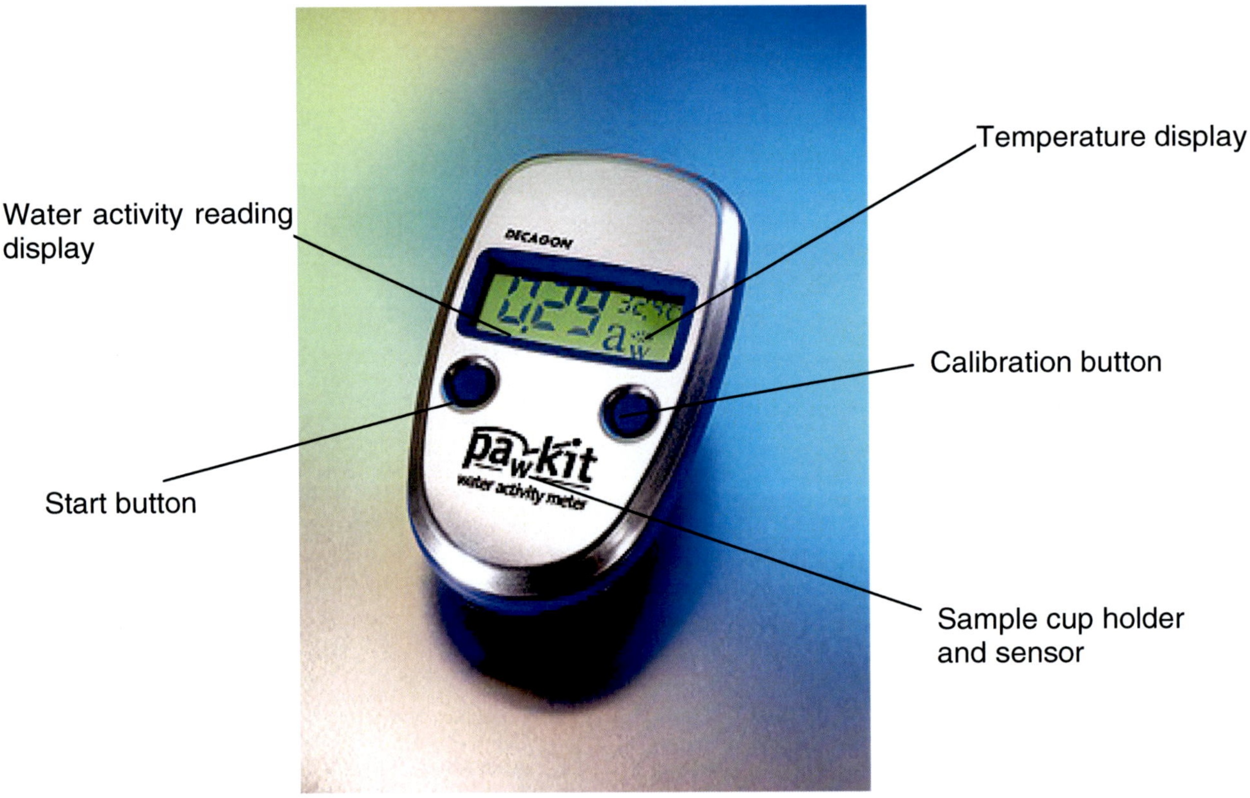

Water activity reading display

Temperature display

Calibration button

Start button

Sample cup holder and sensor

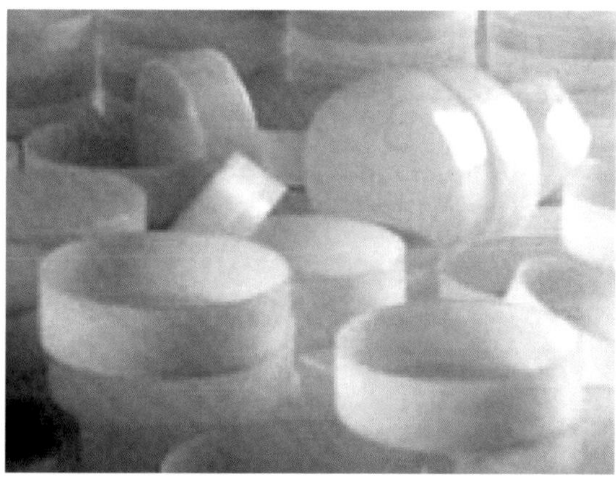

Figure 3. Sample Cups for Pawkit

6.9   Significance of Expiry Dates

All sterilised or disinfected tissues, or consumables and equipment, will be issued with an expiry date. The justification for this expiry date may be based on deterioration of the product or the packaging over time, depending on the storage conditions as specified (for example) in the *Guidelines for the Blood Transfusion Services* in the United Kingdom (9) ('Red Book'), or with tissue grafts it may be based on 'expiry' of the original donor screening process; donor screening and selection processes evolve constantly over time, to incorporate current knowledge and best practice. These may be major changes, such as the introduction of a new mandatory marker, or more minor changes. Minor changes can accumulate to the extent that the selection and screening process changes significantly over time.

6.10 Suggested Reading

1. Bienek C *et al.* Development of a bacteriophage model system to investigate virus inactivation methods used in the treatment of bone allografts. Cell Tissue Bank. 2006. Epub ahead of print.

2. Eagle MJ *et al.* Validation of radiation dose received by frozen unprocessed and processed bone during terminal sterilisation. Cell Tissue Bank 6:221-30 (2005)

3. Grieb TA *et al.* Effective use of optimized, high-dose (50 kGy) gamma irradiation for pathogen inactivation of human bone allografts. Biomaterials 26:2033-42 (2005)

4. Lomas RJ *et al.* Assessment of the biological properties of human split skin allografts disinfected with peracetic acid and preserved in glycerol. Burns. 29:515-25 (2003)

5. Lomas RJ *et al.* Effects of a peracetic acid disinfection protocol on the biocompatibility and biomechanical properties of human patellar tendon allografts. Cell Tissue Bank. 5:149-60 (2004)

6. Pruss A et al. Peracetic acid-ethanol treatment of allogeneic avital bone tissue transplants – a reliable sterilization method. Ann Transplant 8(2):34-42 (2003)

7. Pruss A *et al.* Validation of the 'Marburg bone bank system' for thermodisinfection of allogeneic femoral head transplants using selected bacteria, fungi and spores. Biologicals 31:287-94 (2003)

8. Pruss A *et al.* Validation of the sterilization procedure of allogeneic avital bone transplants using peracetic acid-ethanol. Biologicals. 29:59-66 (2001)

9. Rules and Guidance for Pharmaceutical Manufacturers and Distributors, 7th Edition. Medicines and Healthcare Regulatory Authority. Pharmaceutical Press, 2007. http://www.mhra.gov.uk/Publications/Regulatoryguidance/Medicines/CON2030291

10. Guidelines for the Blood Transfusion Services in the UK, 7th Edition. The Stationary office, London, 2005. http://www.transfusionguidelines.org.uk/Index.aspx?Publication=RB&Section=25&pageid=523

6.11 Self Assessment Questions

Multiple Choice Questions

1. Which of the following decontamination techniques is NOT a sterilisation protocol with regard to vegetative bacteria?
   a. Autoclaving
   b. Ethylene oxide
   c. Antibiotic decontamination
   d. Gamma irradiation
   e. Pasteurisation

2. What concentration hydrogen peroxide is used to process bone allografts?
   a. 0.1%
   b. 1%
   c. 3%
   d. 10%
   e. 30%

3. Which of the following statements is NOT true with regard to glutaradehyde?
   a. It is carcinogenic
   b. Its mode of action is the crosslinking of proteins
   c. Tissues treated with glutaraldehyde are prone to calcify *in vivo*
   d. It is not suitable for the inactivation of viruses
   e. It is widely used in tissue banking

4. Which radioactive isotope is most commonly used in gamma irradiation sterilisation?
   a. Cobalt 60
   b. Polonium 210
   c. Uranium 235
   d. Strontium 90
   e. Carbon 14

Short Answer Questions

1. What factors must be considered when selecting a decontamination protocol for a tissue graft?
2. What types of tissue grafts is ethylene oxide considered suitable as a sterilisation technique?

Assignments

1. You have been asked by a surgeon to recommend a suitable decontamination process for arteries and veins. It is of paramount importance that the structure of the blood vessels and the viability of the cells in the vessels is maintained. What decontamination do you recommend, and why?

2. A patient requires an irradiated bone allograft, but is reluctant to consent to the operation because he thinks that 'radioactive bone will give him cancer'. How would you explain to him that this is not the case?

7   CRYOPRESERVATION

7.1   Introduction

The objective of cryopreservation is to minimise damage to biological materials, including tissues and mammalian cells, during low temperature freezing and storage.

A basic principle of cryopreservation is that the extent of freezing damage depends on the amount of free water in the system and the ability of that water to crystallise during freezing. Water is the major component of all living cells and must be present for chemical reactions to occur within a cell. During freezing, most of the water changes to ice and cellular metabolism ceases.

Ice formation initiates in the extracellular environment, resulting in increased salt concentrations as water is removed to form ice. This ice formation results in an osmotic imbalance. Water then leaves the cells by osmosis and cellular dehydration results. Excessive dehydration can be detrimental to cell recovery.

In 1949, Polge, Smith and Parkes discovered that spermatozoa would survive freezing at −80°C if they were suspended in a saline solution containing glycerol. Six years later, Barnes and Loutit showed that a similar technique could be used to preserve mouse haematopoietic stem cells and that such cryopreserved cells could then be used to rescue animals that had been exposed to a lethal dose of ionising radiation. Lovelock and Bishop introduced dimethyl sulphoxide (DMSO) as an alternative cryoprotectant in 1959, its advantages over glycerol being more rapid diffusion and hence less osmotic stress upon cells. In general, DMSO is the preferred cryoprotectant.

7.2   Variables in Cryopreservation

Cryopreservation is a complex interaction between cryoprotectant, cooling rate, storage temperature and thawing rate and the successful application, for a given cell type or tissue, depends on the optimisation of these variables.

7.2.1   Cryoprotectant

Penetrating cryoprotective agents act by reducing the salt concentration that otherwise increases during the freezing process and because the cryoprotectant is present inside as well as outside the cells they control both intracellular and extracellular salinity. Non-penetrating solutes (such as hydroxyethyl, starch or sucrose) can also have cryoprotective effects but in most applications they are less effective than penetrating cryoprotective agents. They also control the build-up of extracellular salinity but have no effect on intracellular salt concentration.

Cryobiologists use a variety of procedures experimentally to optimise the choice and addition of a cryoprotectant. The method for adding and removing the cryoprotectant needs to be established so that cells are not subjected to serious osmotic stress. This involves measurements to ascertain an estimate of the cell's equilibrium response to changes in external osmolality and the extent to which the cell can be swollen or shrunken without damage. The next step is to consider the kinetics of permeation of the cryoprotectant into the cells and the intrinsic toxicity of the cryoprotectant. Arnaud and Pegg, 1990, showed that the relevant parameters – hydraulic conductivity, solute permeability and solute reflection coefficient can be determined by measuring the time course of change in cell volume in response to a step change in solution composition.

They explained that this should, ideally, be done at a number of temperatures so that toxicity can be determined after equivalent exposure times at each selected temperature. These will not be the same because diffusion is slower at lower temperatures and the required times of exposure are therefore longer. This is, to some degree, countered by the fact that cooling in general reduces toxicity. If an empirical approach is being followed it may be wiser to use a temperature of 0-4°C both for addition and removal of cryoprotectant.

It is essential to determine the optimal concentration of cryoprotectant to minimise the known toxic effects of the compound. This can be achieved by exposing cells to increasing concentrations of cryoprotectant at a set temperature, e.g. 0-4°C, for a fixed time, e.g. 30 mins and then removing the cryoprotectant by a decreasing sequence of concentration steps. An appropriate functional assay can then be used to determine the optimal concentration of cryoprotectant for a given cell or tissue type.

7.2.2   Cooling Rate

The optimal cooling rate for cells and tissues will be defined by the rate that permits some cell shrinkage without the formation of significant amounts of intracellular ice. Tolerances for cell shrinkage and intracellular ice formation vary between cell and tissue types. The effects of cooling rate and concentration of cryoprotectant interact. Cooling rates that are too slow increase the length of time that cells are exposed to the cryoprotectant at the higher temperatures. This can lead to significant toxicity. In contrast, where cooling rates are too high, the cryoprotectant is unable to enter the cells rapidly enough to prevent the nucleation of ice crystals inside the cells, leading to cell death.

With many cell types a concentration of 1 to 2M DMSO (1.3M = 10% w/v) and a cooling rate of 1°C/min has shown to be optimal but it is advisable when establishing a new protocol to perform validation to determine optimal rates to achieve better functional survival.

7.2.3   Storage Temperature

Although temperatures below - 80°C can be used for relatively short periods of time, up to 6 months, a storage temperature of - 150 to - 180°C is recommended for the storage of products for clinical use. Procedures must be in place to avoid significant warming of stored product during the addition/removal of other units of cells. Above the glass transition point (circa -135°C) there is still free water in the system which is in dynamic equilibrium with the frozen water (ice). Therefore some new ice crystals are forming as others melt. There is a risk that the new crystals will form inside the cells and hence kill the cells. Therefore there is a very slow but progressive loss of viability through time. Once below the glass transition temperature, all of the water is immobilised and hence new ice crystals do not form.

7.2.4   Thawing Rate

For most cell types rapid thawing, by immersion in a 37°C water/saline bath will be optimal and is essential for cells cooled rapidly to avoid the growth of intracellular ice formed during the freezing process.

7.2.5   Dilution of Cryoprotectant

Cryoprotectant, at a concentration of 10% at normothermic temperatures, will be toxic to cells. It is therefore necessary to dilute the concentration to a level below which the toxic effect is removed. This is essential for cells that will be cultured for a period of time after thawing. The method should be designed for slow dilution over 10 –15 mins (Figure 1). The cell suspension will then, usually, be centrifuged and the cells re-suspended in appropriate medium.

This procedure is not without its risks and must be carried out with care to avoid damaging the cells which may still be fragile following the thawing procedure.

For some cells such as bone marrow and peripheral blood stem cells there are divided opinions as to the virtue of including a dilution step since there will be an adequate dilution when re-implanted.

Figure 1. Cryopreservation of Stem Cells

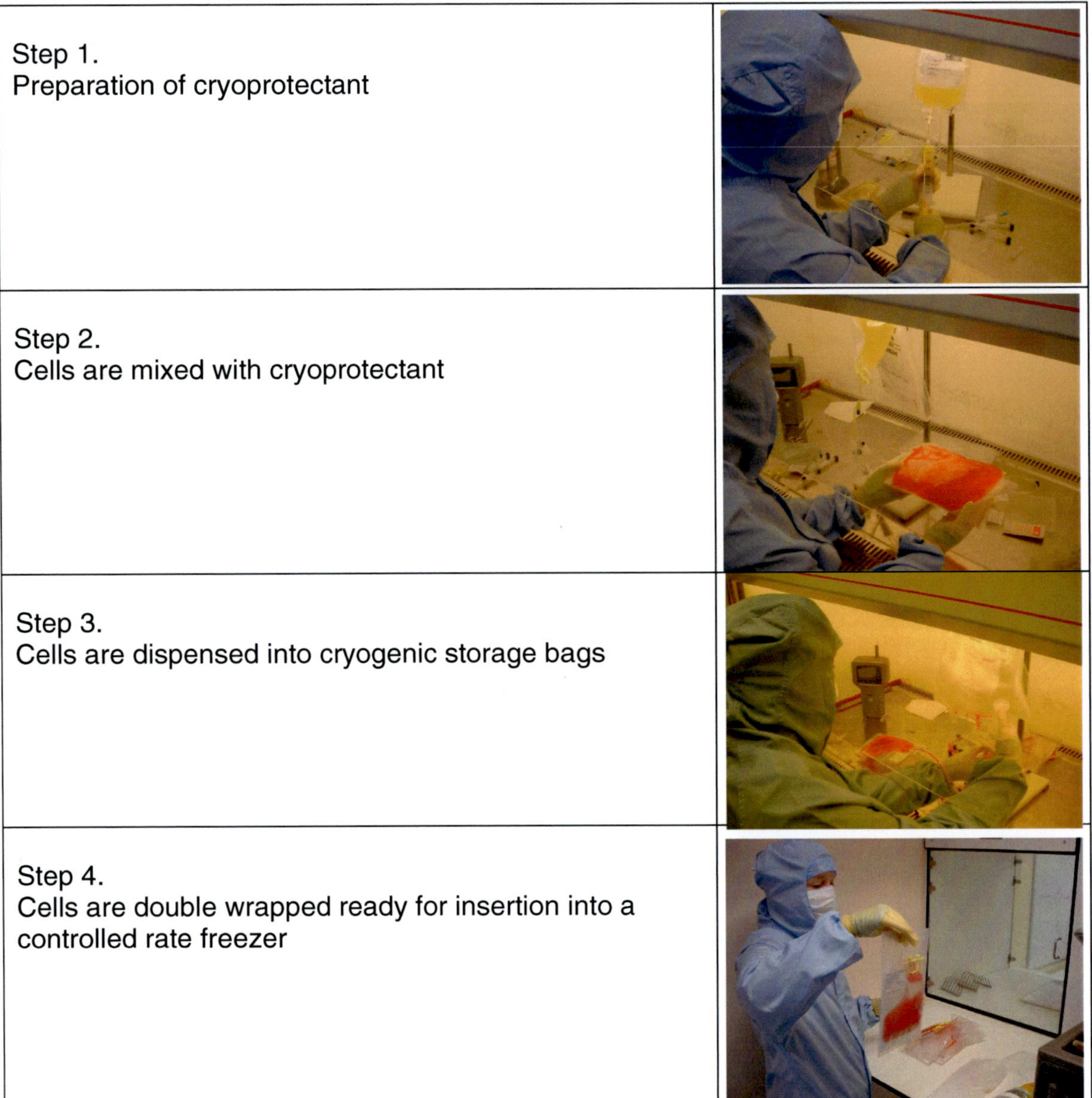

Step 1. Preparation of cryoprotectant	
Step 2. Cells are mixed with cryoprotectant	
Step 3. Cells are dispensed into cryogenic storage bags	
Step 4. Cells are double wrapped ready for insertion into a controlled rate freezer	

7.2.6   Controlled Rate Freezing

The advantage of using a controlled rate freezer over a non-automated procedure for cooling cell suspensions is that it provides for a reproducible method of freezing each time the procedure is carried out. It is also possible to programme variable rates of cooling at different points during the procedure. Also it is possible to include into the cooling programme a step which will initiate freezing of the sample and also compensate for the latent heat that is released as the cell suspension freezes. This is achieved by including a rapid rate of cooling at the theoretical freezing point of the suspension before returning to the desired cooling rate.

Controlled rate freezers operate by injecting, into the freezing chamber, an amount of liquid nitrogen which may be determined by a temperature sensor controlling the chamber or the sample itself and comparing this to the temperature required by the set programme. The admission of liquid nitrogen is controlled by the opening and closing of a solenoid valve in response to the need for liquid nitrogen. The controlled rate freezers will have some form of device to provide a record of the cooling run in addition to alarms to indicate when the cooling rate has deviated from the desired set rate.

7.2.7   Transport of Frozen Product

It is important to ensure that the product remains frozen during transport to the unit where it will be thawed and used.

If it is certain that the product will be used within a short period of time after delivery and that the total storage time will be short then material can be transported at −80°C by using solid carbon dioxide (cardice) within an insulated container. It is important to use a container that has been validated to ensure that there will be sufficient cardice to last for the entire storage period. The procedure must be validated to show that the storage container is not permeable to carbon dioxide to avoid possible contact between the gas and product.

If the product has been stored under the surface of liquid nitrogen, a practice that is not normally recommended due to the known possible risks of cross contamination, then it is possible to transport the product in an insulated container with liquid nitrogen. Again, it is important to carry out a validation to ensure that there will be sufficient liquid nitrogen for the entire transport time. This method is very hazardous due to the possibility of spillage of liquid nitrogen and is really only suitable for transport over very short distances. Care must be taken to avoid the risks associated with liquid nitrogen such as spillages and asphyxiation. The use of containers with liquid nitrogen is not allowed on airlines and is very dangerous when used unattended in a car.

Dry shippers are designed to safely transport cryopreserved products at temperatures of around −190°C. These are mobile, insulated containers that contain a material that is porous to liquid nitrogen and capable of holding very low temperatures usually for a couple of weeks. This means that there is no actual liquid within the container when fully primed. It is essential that the dry shipper is validated to confirm what the holding time is at temperatures of −190°C and below. When the temperature rises above this level, the temperature rise will become very rapid and it is an indication that the shipper will require re-charging with fresh liquid nitrogen. It is important that a logbook is kept which details when the shipper has been re-charged. Care must be taken since a freshly charged shipper will contain liquid in the transport chamber until it has been fully absorbed. Temperature loggers are available for fitting to the lid of dry shippers to enable the user to monitor the temperature within the chamber during transport.

7.3   Packaging for Storage and Handling Frozen Products

There are some considerations that must be taken into account when selecting a container for freezing cells. Plastic is preferred to glass as it is less likely to shatter at the extreme temperature of storage. However, a full validation must be carried out to ensure that the container is suitable for storage at low temperatures and also that the rates of cooling of the product can be achieved.

When the product is of human origin or another source of potentially hazardous material then it is essential that the product is stored also within a secondary container. This is to avoid the possibility of cross contamination between stored units. This risk can arise during processing or during storage of the product.

Regardless of the type of container chosen it will be very fragile at the low storage temperatures of −150 to −180°C and care must be taken when handling frozen product to avoid the possibility of damage to the container and ultimately to loss of product upon thawing. Care must be taken in choosing an appropriate inventory system for the type of packaging used. It is important to discuss, fully, with the supplier of storage refrigerators, your inventory requirements. They should be designed so that the entire contents of the package sit within the height of the inventory container. Care should also be taken to avoid overpacking within a storage area since damage to the package can occur during removal from storage. When product is stored in plastic bags, consideration should be given to placing bags from one collection in a cardboard outer box to provide protection from possible mechanical damage. In any event, if transporting stored material in dry shippers between Centres, it is advisable to place units in an outer wrapping such as cardboard since movement of the frozen units within the 'shipper' will increase the risk of damage.

7.3.1   Safety in Handling Liquid Nitrogen

When handled with due care and attention, liquid nitrogen is perfectly safe. However, as a very cold liquid, with a boiling point of −196°C it can be extremely hazardous if mishandled.

The risks associated with burns injuries can be brought about by not using appropriate personal protective clothing such as face covering, insulated gloves and long sleeved clothing. It is not advisable to wear open toed sandals when working with liquid nitrogen. Care must be taken to ensure that items of clothing do not provide potential pockets for liquid nitrogen to get trapped.

Nitrogen gas cannot be detected by human senses as it is colourless, odourless and tasteless. Breathing an atmosphere that contains less than 18% oxygen can cause dizziness and quickly lead to unconsciousness and death. It is, therefore, very important to ensure that rooms, where liquid nitrogen is being used, or stored, are continually monitored and alarmed to detect low levels of oxygen.

Improperly sealed containers, that have been stored immersed in liquid nitrogen, may explode on removal from storage. It is best to avoid the use of glass ampoules. Overtightening the lids on plastic vials can result in damage to the seal and result in leakage if samples are stored 'under liquid nitrogen'.

It is important to only use containers that are designed for liquid nitrogen; not all dewar flasks are intended for this purpose. The user should also ensure that containers, used to transport liquid nitrogen or samples in vapour phase nitrogen, are not sealed and thereby preventing nitrogen gas from venting.

7.4   Suggested Reading

1. Polge C. et al. Revival of spermatozoa after vitrification and dehydration at low temperatures. Nature, 164: 666 (1949)

2. Lovelock JE. The mechanism of the protective action of glycerol against haemolysis by freezing and thawing. Biochim. Biophys. Acta. 11:28-36, (1953)

3. Mazur P. Kinetics of water loss from cells at subzero temperatures and the likelihood of intracellular freezing. J Gen Phvsiol. 47: 347-369 (1963)

4. Song YC. et al. Cryopreservation of the common carotid artery of the rabbit: Optimization of dimethyl sulphoxide concentration and cooling rate. Cryobiology, 32:405-421 (1995)

5. Hunt CJ, et al. Cryopreservation of umbilical cord blood: 1. Osmotically inactive volume, hydraulic conductivity and permeability of $CD34^+$ cells to dimethyl sulphoxide. Cryobiology, 46:61-75 (2003).

6. Pegg DE. The preservation of tissues for transplantation. Cell and Tissue Banking. 7:349-358 (2006).

7. Society for Low Temperature Biology. www.sltb.info

8. Society for Cryobiology. www.societyforcryobiology.org

7.5   Self Assessment Questions

Multiple Choice Questions

1. The optimal final concentration of DMSO for cryopreservation of stem cells is approximately:
   a) 0.1%
   b) 1.0%
   c) 10%
   d) 25%
   e) 50%

2. The optimal freezing rate for cryopreservation of stem cells is approximately:
   a) 0.1°C/minute
   b) -1°C/minute
   c) -5°C/minute
   d) -10°C/minute
   e) -1°C/hour

3. Which of the following may be used as a cryoprotectant?
   a) Glycerol
   b) Dimethyl sulphoxide
   c) Hydroxyethyl starch
   d) Potassium chloride
   e) Aluminium hydroxide

4. Liquid nitrogen has a boiling point of:
   a) -150°C
   b) -190°C
   c) -196°C
   d) -80°C
   e) -96°C

Short Answer Questions

1. Why is it important to control cooling rate during cryopreservation?

Assignments

1. Prepare an outline specification for a cryogenic storage facility which will use liquid nitrogen. Which features are intended to protect staff from health and safety risks associated with the use of liquid nitrogen?

2. Discuss the advantages and disadvantages of vapour-phase nitrogen storage compared to liquid nitrogen phase storage.

8 STEM CELL BIOLOGY

8.1 Terminology

A stem cell is a special kind of cell that has a unique capacity to renew itself and to give rise to defined cell types. Chapter 4 provides an overview of haematopoietic stem cells. Although most cells of the body, such as those of the heart or skin, are committed to conduct a specific function, a stem cell is uncommitted and remains uncommitted, until it receives a signal to develop into a specialised cell. Their proliferative capacity combined with the ability to become specialised makes stem cells unique. This ability has encouraged scientists for many years to look for ways to use stem cells to replace cells and tissues that are damaged or diseased.

Stem cells may be derived from the embryo, foetus or adult and although these cells all share many characteristics there are also some important differences. It is essential to use clearly defined terminology when discussing stem cells and so a list of key definitions follows.

8.1.1 Embryonic Stem Cell

An embryonic stem cell is derived from a group of cells called the inner cell mass, which is part of the early (4- to 5-day) embryo called the blastocyst. Once removed from the blastocyst, the cells of the inner cell mass can be cultured into embryonic stem cells and encouraged to proliferate indefinitely. Much basic understanding about embryonic stem cells has come from animal research. Embryonic stem cells are not themselves embryos and do not necessarily behave in the laboratory as they would in the developing embryo.

8.1.2 Embryonic Germ Cell

An embryonic germ cell is derived from foetal tissue. Specifically, they are isolated from the primordial germ cells of the gonadal ridge of the 5- to 10-week foetus. Later in development, the gonadal ridge develops into the testes or ovaries and the primordial germ cells give rise to eggs or sperm. Embryonic stem cells and embryonic germ cells are not identical in their properties and characteristics.

8.1.3 Pluripotent Stem Cell

A single pluripotent stem cell has the ability to give rise to types of cells that develop from the three germ layers (mesoderm, endoderm, and ectoderm) from which all the cells of the body arise. Human pluripotent stem cells have been isolated and cultured from early human embryos and from foetal tissue that was destined to be part of the gonads. It is not clear whether truly pluripotent stem cells can be isolated from adult tissue.

8.1.4 Adult Stem Cell

An adult stem cell is an undifferentiated (unspecialised) cell that occurs in a differentiated (specialised) tissue, renews itself, and becomes specialised to yield all of the specialised cell types of the tissue from which it originated. Adult stem cells are capable of making identical copies of themselves for the lifetime of the organism. This property is referred to as "self-renewal." Adult stem cells usually divide to generate progenitor or precursor cells, which then differentiate or develop into "mature" cell types that have characteristic shapes and specialised functions, e.g., muscle cell contraction or nerve cell signalling. Sources of adult stem cells include bone marrow, blood, the cornea and the retina of the eye, brain, skeletal muscle, dental pulp, liver, skin, the lining of the gastrointestinal tract, and pancreas. The most abundant information about adult human stem cells comes from studies of haematopoietic (blood-forming) stem cells isolated from the bone marrow and blood.

These adult stem cells have been extensively studied and applied therapeutically for various diseases. At this point, there is no isolated population of adult stem cells that is capable of forming all the kinds of cells of the body. Adult stem cells are rare. Often they are difficult to identify, isolate, and purify.

8.1.5   Progenitor Cells

A progenitor cell occurs in fetal or adult tissues and is partially specialised; it divides and gives rise to differentiated cells. Researchers often distinguish progenitor cells from adult stem cells in the following way: when a stem cell divides, one of the two new cells is often a stem cell capable of replicating itself again. In contrast, when a progenitor cell divides, it can form more progenitor cells or it can form two specialised cells, neither of which is capable of replicating itself. Progenitor cells can replace cells that are damaged or dead, thus maintaining the integrity and functions of a tissue such as liver or brain. Progenitor cells give rise to related types of cells e.g. lymphocytes such as T cells, B cells and natural killer cells but in their normal state do not generate a wide variety of cell types.

8.1.6   Plasticity

Plasticity is the ability of an adult stem cell from one tissue to generate the specialised cell type(s) of another tissue. An example of plasticity is that, under specific experimental conditions, adult stem cells from bone marrow can generate cells that resemble neurons and other cell types that are commonly found in the brain. The concept of adult stem cell plasticity is new, and the phenomenon is not thoroughly understood. Evidence suggests that, given the right environment, some adult stem cells are capable of being "genetically reprogrammed" to generate specialised cells that are characteristic of different tissues.

8.1.7   Differentiation

Differentiation is the process by which an unspecialised cell (such as a stem cell) becomes specialised into one of the many cells that make up the body. During differentiation, certain genes become activated and other genes become inactivated in an intricately regulated way. As a result, a differentiated cell develops specific structures and performs certain functions. For example, a mature, differentiated nerve cell has thin, fiber-like projections that send and receive the electrochemical signals that permit the nerve cell to communicate with other nerve cells. In the laboratory, a stem cell can be manipulated to become specialised or partially specialised cell types (e.g., heart muscle, nerve, or pancreatic cells) and this is known as directed differentiation.

8.2   Comparisons of Adult Stem Cells and Embryonic Stem Cells

Are human adult and embryonic stem cells equivalent in their potential for generating replacement cells and tissues? Current science indicates that, although both of these cell types hold enormous promise, adult and embryonic stem cells differ in important ways. What is not known is the extent to which these different cell types will be useful for the development of cell-based therapies to treat disease.

8.2.1 How are Adult and Embryonic Stem Cells Similar?

In most cases, stem cells can be isolated and maintained in an unspecialised state. Scientists use similar techniques (i.e. cell-surface markers and monitoring the expression of certain genes) to identify or characterise stem cells as being unspecialised. Scientists then use different genetic or molecular markers to determine that the cells have differentiated—a process that might be compared to distinguishing a particular cell type by reading its cellular barcode. Stem cells from both adult and embryonic sources can proliferate and specialise when transplanted into an animal with a compromised immune system. (Immune-deficient animals are less likely to reject the transplanted tissue). Scientists also have evidence that differentiated cells generated from either stem cell type undergo "homing," a process whereby the transplanted cells are attracted by and travel to a site of injury. Similarly, researchers are finding that the cellular and noncellular "environment" into which stem cell derived tissues are placed, whether they are grown in a culture dish or transplanted into an animal, greatly influences how the cells differentiate.

8.2.2 How are Adult and Embryonic Stem Cells Different?

Perhaps the most distinguishing feature of embryonic stem cells and adult stem cells is their source. Most scientists now agree that adult stem cells exist in many tissues of the human body (in vivo), although the cells are quite rare. In contrast, it is less certain that embryonic stem cells exist as such in the embryo. Instead, embryonic stem cells develop in tissue culture after they are derived from the inner cell mass of the early embryo.

Depending on the culture conditions, embryonic stem cells may form clumps of cells that can differentiate spontaneously to generate many cell types. This property has not been observed in cultures of adult stem cells. Also, if undifferentiated embryonic stem cells are removed from the culture dish and injected into a mouse with a compromised immune system, a benign tumour called a teratoma can develop. A teratoma typically contains a mixture of partially differentiated cell types. For this reason, scientists do not anticipate that undifferentiated embryonic stem cells will be used for transplants or other therapeutic applications. Stem cells in adult tissues do not appear to have the same capacity to differentiate as embryonic stem cells.

Embryonic stem are clearly pluripotent; they can differentiate into any tissues derived from all three germ layers of the embryo (ectoderm, mesoderm, and endoderm). But are adult stem cells also pluripotent? When they reside in their normal tissue compartments—the brain, the bone marrow, the epithelial lining of the gut, etc.— they produce the cells that are specific to that kind of tissue and they have been found in tissues derived from all three embryonic layers. However it has not yet been shown that a single adult stem cell can give rise to specialised cells derived from all three embryonic germ cell layers. Therefore, a single adult stem cell has not been shown to have the same degree of pluripotency as embryonic stem cells.

8.3 Pluripotent versus Multipotent Stem Cells

The stem cell compartment can be arbitrarily divided into two: embryonic stem (ES) cells and "tissue specific" or "adult" stem cells. The former are pluripotent and are able to generate most tissue types in an organism. These cells may be regarded as truly 'plastic' in their developmental potential. In contrast, 'adult or tissue specific' stem cells have been used in clinical settings for haematological disorders for many years and are often multipotent, giving rise to many lineages, particularly those in the tissue within which they arise. General experimental approaches and paradigms applicable to adult or tissue specific mammalian stem cells were defined first in the haematopoietic system.

Therefore, the haematopoietic stem cell (HSC) is the best characterised adult mammalian stem cell type, and has been used to establish the criteria for defining stemness of cells in other mammalian adult tissues.

8.4   Defining the Haematopoietic Stem Cells

HSC are defined by their capacity to repopulate the whole haematopoietic system. This has been proven *in vivo* in mice by transplantation of single stem cells into syngeneic animals, in non-human primate studies and following transplantation for haematological diseases in humans. Surrogate *in vivo* animal models of human haematopoiesis include the use of SCID, NOD/SCID, beige-nude-SCID (bnx), Rag-1 deficient/NOD, nude/NOD/SCID and β2-microglobulin deficient NOD/SCID mice to measure human SCID repopulating cells (SCR) from haematopoietic tissues. An alternative is the *in utero* transplantation of human cells into sheep. None of these surrogate models shows full human donor derived haematopoiesis *in vivo* but, depending on the system used, they contribute to a proportion of or most haematopoietic lineages. Thus, successful long-term transplantation of human stem cells into patients with haematological malignancies or genetic diseases, which was introduced in 1968, remains the gold standard for transplantation for other diseases. More than 50,000 transplants per annum are now carried out world-wide, with more than 20,000 in Europe. In this setting, both autologous and allogeneic (identical twin, HLA-matched sibling, other family members, HLA-matched unrelated donors) transplants are performed (see Chapter 4).

8.5   The Properties of Haematopoietic Stem Cells

There are three major properties that identify the HSC and that have been used to analyse other tissue specific stem cells. First, although HSCs are rare, occurring with a frequency of around 1 in 10^4 to 10^5 total bone marrow nucleated cells, they have an extensive proliferative capacity and the ability to balance 'self-renewal' and differentiation, ensuring a sustained population within the bone marrow, where the microenvironmental niche regulates their fate. Second, they are multipotent and clonogenic (i.e. a single cell can give rise to ten to eleven functional committed haematopoietic cell lineages) over an individual life span (Figure 1). Thirdly, they are quiescent or slowly cycling. Thus, HSCs have, for many years, been considered to be 'plastic' in their abilities to regulate the balance between maintaining the stem cell compartment and providing sufficient progeny to meet the demands required to produce over one billion blood cells per day under normal homeostatic conditions or to generate specific subsets of haematopoietic cells during times of haematological stress. Murine HSCs have been purified to near-homogeneity, and this has allowed their *in vitro* and *in vivo* analysis at a single or clonal cell level. In most mammalian species, the enriched HSCs are heterogeneous, and practically the HSC compartment encompasses cells with differing proliferative or self-renewing potentials, i.e. it contains a continuum of stem cell types.

Figure 1. Schematic Representation of the Hierarchy of Haematopoietic Development.

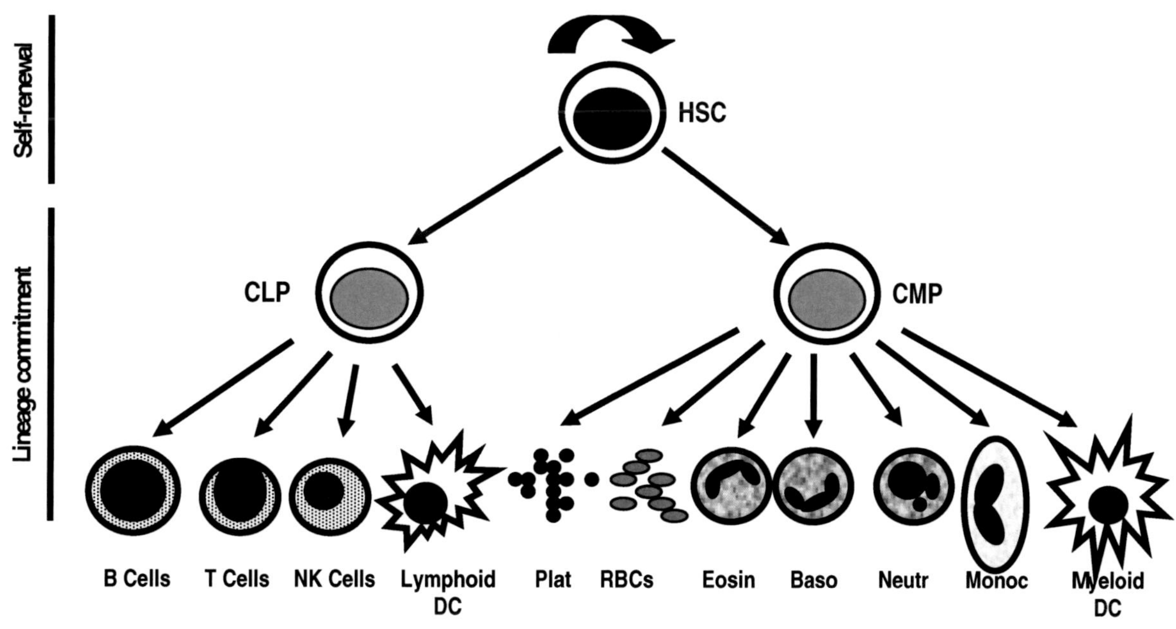

Key.

A haematopoietic stem cell (HSC) balances self-renewal with lineage commitment and differentiation, giving rise to more HSCs and differentiated blood components, that is, myeloid and lymphoid lineages. CLP, common lymphoid progenitor; CMP, common myeloid progenitor; B cells, B-lymphocytes; T cells, T-lymphocytes; NK cells, natural killer cells, Lymphoid DC, lymphoid dendritic cell; Plat, platelets; RBCs, red blood cells; Eosin, eosinophils; Baso, basophils; Neutr, neutrophils; Monoc, monocytes and Myeloid DC, myeloid dendritic cells.

8.6   Stem Cell Plasticity or Potentiality?

More recent studies on stem cells derived from haematopoietic and other tissues have led to newer concepts of stem cell plasticity or potentiality. These relate to the ability of a stem cell or a more mature cell (i) to apparently switch or generate additional unexpected lineages and acquire the phenotype of a stem cell from a different tissue or organ (Figure 2), and (ii) in some cases to cross embryological determined boundaries i.e. to switch between somatic mesodermal, ectodermal and endodermal lineages. Thus, exploiting adult stem cell plasticity or potentiality beyond the haematopoietic system may be useful for regenerative medicine.

There is a heterogeneous group of human diseases, such as neurodegenerative and cardiovascular diseases, cancer, etc., for which stem cell-based knowledge and therapies might be particularly beneficial and of immediate use therapeutically. There are five pathways that have been used to explain these newer concepts of "stem cell plasticity" or potentiality (Figure 2), although detailed mechanisms are not yet understood. The first is the **dedifferentiation** of a mature or lineage restricted cell to a more immature progenitor or precursor cell, followed by differentiation to another lineage. The second is **transdetermination**: the situation in which stem cell potential is redirected giving rise to cell types of a different stem/precursor cell. The third pathway to a new identity is **transdifferentiation**, the mechanism by which a differentiated cell can gain the phenotypic characteristics of another differentiated cell. The fourth pathway that could explain cell plasticity occurs via **cell fusion**.

Finally, an alternative explanation is that certain tissues contain **very primitive** or **multiple stem cell** types, the potential of which is expressed when the stem cell enters and interacts with an appropriate and specific microenvironment.

It may be possible to reprogramme haematopoietic stem cells or stem cells from different sources by the process of nuclear reprogramming, but the usefulness in transplantation awaits further experimentation.

Figure 2. Pathways to New Identities

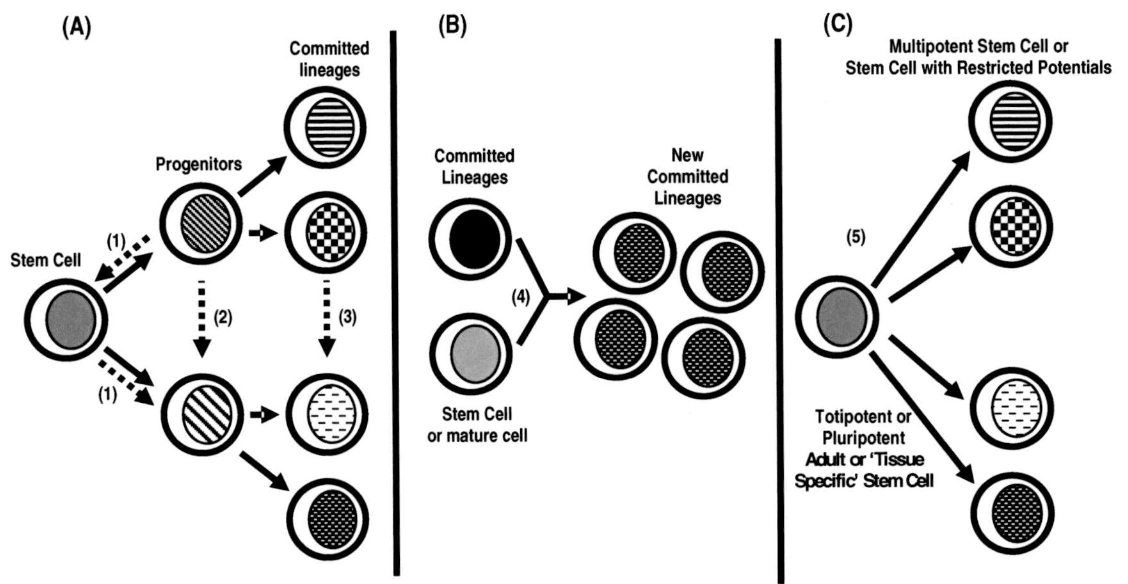

Key.
Traditionally, a hierarchical model of cell differentiation has been accepted. Totipotent, pluripotent or multipotent stem cells give rise to progenitor cells that gradually differentiate into committed cell lineages. Recently, the concept of stem cell plasticity has been proposed. The underlying mechanisms by which a stem/progenitor or more mature cell acquires the phenotype of another cell type are not yet understood. However, the pathways to new cell identities may be explained by the following processes: (1) dedifferentiation, followed by differentiation into different lineage, (2) transdetermination, (3) transdifferentiation, (4) cell fusion and (5) a totipotent or pluripotent stem cell gives rise to a multipotent stem cell or a stem cell with restricted potentials. A potential illustration of dedifferentiation is seen after limb amputation in newts, where myocytes can generate cells of different lineages. An example of possible transdetermination occurs when cells are transplanted between imaginal discs in the *Drosophila* larvae. Generally, the transplanted cells maintain their own identity, but some of them gain the identity of the new location. There are indications of transdifferentiation occurring during normal development when smooth muscle cells give rise to skeletal myocytes in the oesophagus. Finally, an experimental example of cell fusion has been demonstrated with therapeutic cloning, where a mature lineage restricted cell nucleus can be reprogrammed by its insertion into an enucleated ovum.

8.7 Stem Cells in Haematopoietic Tissues

8.7.1 Haematopoietic Stem Cells

Although the potentiality of stem cells derived from haematopoietic tissues has been accepted for a long time, the newer concepts of adult stem cell plasticity remain controversial. This is because it is not always established if there are different types of stem cells in different tissues or if a defined stem cell type, such as an HSC can switch lineages. A key issue is to identify the starting cell population or cell subset, and to analyse the designated stem cell at a single cell or clonal level, with a read-out of as many cell types as possible. The identification and purification of human HSCs have shown that repopulating cells belong to the $CD34^+$ and $CD34^-$ cell fraction. They are found postnatally in the bone marrow, umbilical cord blood and non-mobilised or mobilised peripheral blood. These cells lack lineage markers (Lin^-). In the human, they are generally $CD38^-$ and there are indications that $CD34^-$ cells might be more primitive than $CD34^+$ cells. CD133 has also been found on human HSCs and marks a percentage of the $CD34^+$ and $CD34^-$ cells.

Other important surface markers have been identified in or on or used to isolate human or murine stem cell subsets with haematopoietic long-term repopulating potential. Most are not haematopoietic specific and their expression on HSCs is variable. Other studies suggest that aldehyde dehydrogenase may be one of the fewer reliable markers for HSC isolation in rodents and humans.

8.7.2 Non Haematopoietic Stem Cells in Haematopoietic Tissues

As well as the haematopoietic system, self-renewing adult or tissue specific somatic stem cells have been reported to be maintained in many if not all tissues. Such adult stem cells serve to replace the differentiated cells in the case of injury or stress to the tissue or when there is a constant need to replenish mature cells (e.g. blood and skin). In recent years, scientists have provided evidence that stem cells in haematopoietic and non-haematopoietic tissues have the potential to generate cell types other than those of the tissue in which they reside.

Haematopoietic tissues or organs, such as bone marrow, are thought to contain at least three primitive stem/progenitor cell subset as well as haematopoietic stem cells and references therein). However, stem cell potential is defined by and reliant on the readout system or assay and this may provide an inappropriate or minimal calculation of their potentiality. At least three phenotypically distinct stem cell subsets have been identified in haematopoietic tissues. These are (i) the haemangioblast (HB), a precursor of haematopoietic and endothelial stem cells, (ii) mesenchymal stem cells (MSC) that give rise to stroma, pericytes, muscle, bone, cartilage, and fat cells, and (iii) the most recently defined multipotent adult progenitor cells (MAPC) that generate most if not all, ectodermal, endodermal and mesodermal cell lineages. These may or may not fall within the $CD34^+$ cell subset and include precursors for cells that are located, though not exclusively within haematopoietic tissues, e.g. blood vessel endothelia, stromal reticular cells, fat cells and osteoblasts.

8.8   Can Stem Cells From Haematopoietic Tissues Repair Other Damaged Tissues?

Bone marrow transplantation has been successfully practised for over 30 years. Its success has relied on a detailed understanding of the basic biology and regulation of haematopoietic stem cells.

We know from many studies that the HSC has a huge potential, with such cells in bone marrow being able to produce over one billion blood cells per day. We also know how to repair diseased bone marrow and have recommended dosages of CD34+ cells for this repair to be effective. Similar approaches have been applied to skin stem cells and their use in burns patients and MSC are being used to repair bone and cartilage defects, particularly when coupled with cellular scaffolds and bioengineering. Other organ repair systems are more complex and endogenous stem cells in such organs may have a much more restricted proliferative ability, especially in adults.

Those that fall into this category include the heart and brain. Furthermore, damage to the brain or spinal cord will only be repaired with the establishment of the appropriate neural connections. Repair of damage to the heart following myocardial infarction requires revascularisation from endothelial precursors and their associated smooth muscle cells or pericytes, either by transplantation strategies or by reactivating endogenous cells at the site of the infarct. It also requires replacement of damaged cardiomyocytes, which form correct connections and mediate appropriate heart functions. It has been predicted that there are in the order of 2×10^9 cardiomyocytes in the left ventricle of the human heart, and that up to 25% can be damaged in a myocardial infarction. Cardiomyocytes possess a modest capacity to regenerate after injury. There are some reports that they have been derived *in vitro* from MSC and MAPC in haematopoietic organs, although these are controversial. Lately, bone marrow derived cells have been reported to be stimulators of angiogenesis in ischaemic heart disease in humans. Methods include percutaneous delivery of autologous unfractionated cells as a sole therapy, purified bone marrow-derived precursor cells (CD133[+] cells) injected along the infarct zone at the time of coronary artery bypass, and intracoronary infusion of autologous unfractionated progenitor cells. These studies demonstrate that intracardiac injection of cells is feasible and safe. Repair of this damage by transplantation with cardiomyocytes or their precursors derived from haematopoietic or non-haematopoietic tissues at different stages of development, or by stimulation of endogenous cell production are approaches requiring considerable experimentation in animal models of this disease. Long-term clinical outcomes await the results of larger-scale randomised trials, and experimental evidence for the phenotype of injected cells, the timing of the cell therapies and the functional effects in failing heart models are required. Thus, we must understand how to manipulate these cells both *in vitro* and *in vivo*, with particular emphasis on expanding stem or progenitor cell subsets and in generating functionally effective end cells that are of therapeutic usefulness.

8.9   Conclusions

The regulation of the fate of stem cells from haematopoietic tissues is thought to be driven extrinsically, through growth factors, cytokines, stroma or other external cues, and intrinsically, as part of an endogenous programme of differentiation that involves signal transduction pathways.

The areas of prime importance experimentally, that will help in determining stem cell potential, are: (i) to define the molecular signature of the stem cell so that the stem cell and its potentiality can be assessed quickly without the need for long-term repopulation assays; (ii) to expand stem cells, and (iii) to regulate stem cell differentiation so that appropriate functional end cells can be used therapeutically. Some of these issues are now being addressed. We are now at an exciting phase of stem cell research where basic studies will lead to new clinical treatments.

8.10   Further Reading

1.   An overview of stem cell biology
     http://www.facsnet.org/tools/sci_tech/biotek/stem_cell.php3#what
2.   *Thomas' Hematopoietic Cell Transplantation.* Blume KG, Forman SJ, Appelbaum FR (eds). Pages 69 to 95; parts of Sections 5, 6 and 7.

8.11

8.11   Self-Assessment Questions

Short Answer Questions

1. What special characteristics are unique to stem cells?
2. List some tissues which contain adult stem cells.

Assignments

1. Discuss the contention that advances in stem cell biology are taking transplantation medicine from an era of organ replacement to an era of tissue repair.
2. Consider the extent to which scientific studies support the existence of transdifferentiation.

9 BIOLOGY OF SKIN TISSUE

9.1 Structure of Skin

Skin is the largest organ in the body. It fulfils a number of life saving functions, acting as a barrier to the ingress of bacteria into the underlying tissues and preventing the excessive loss of water from the body surface.

Skin comprises of two major layers, the outer epidermis and underlying this is the dermis. Beneath the dermis is the subcutaneous fat (Figure 1).

Figure 1. The Structure of Skin

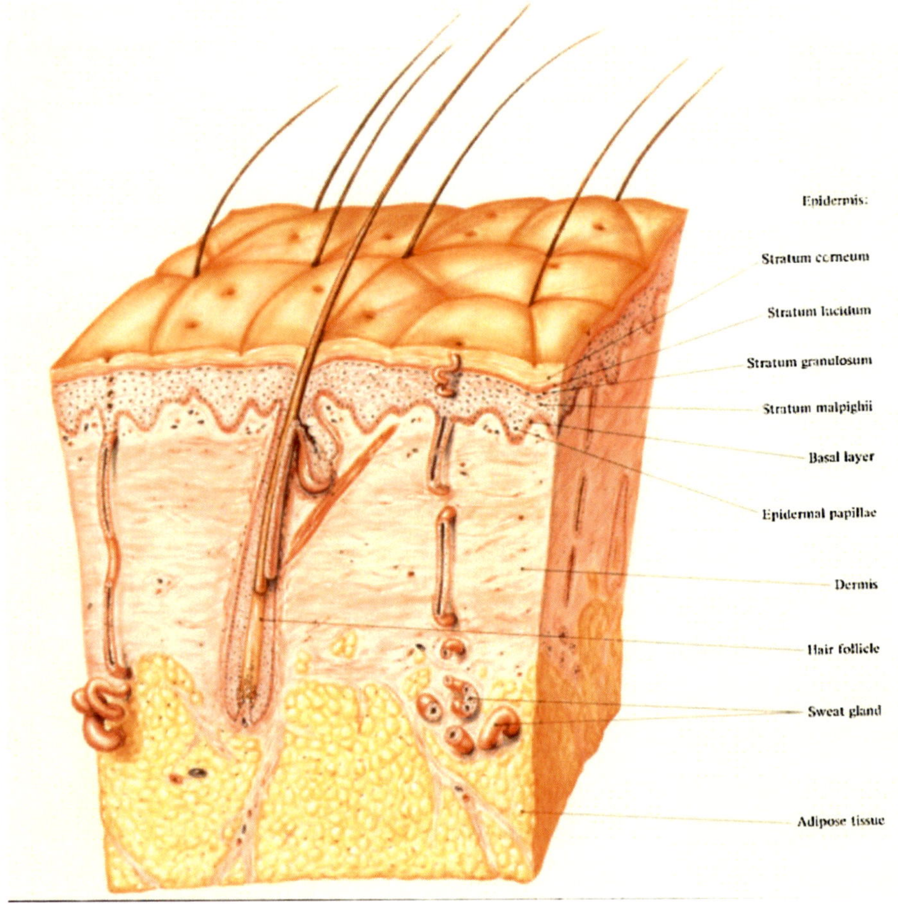

9.1.1 Epidermis

The epidermis is a thin layer only 0.5-1.5mm thick. It comprises of a basement membrane on which are located basal keratinocytes. The basal keratinocytes proliferate continuously by cell division. Some of the basal keratinocytes are stem cells i.e. are immortal cells that continue dividing throughout life. Others are programmed to undergo a finite number of cell divisions. Many daughter cells move off the basement membrane moving towards the surface. Many of these are "transient amplifying cells" that undergo further cell divisions as they move up towards the surface. As they approach the surface the cells die and undergo characteristic changes, becoming flattened and cornified as a result of changes in the keratin proteins within the cells. These outermost cells form a very tough interlocking layer known as the "stratum corneum". It is the stratum corneum that prevents ingress of bacteria and loss of water. In addition to the "stratum corneum" many of the other "strata" or layers within the epidermis are given names to reflect their morphological appearance under the microscope (Figure 1). As keratinocytes move up from the basement membrane, they are cast off or shed from the skin surface. The vast majority of "dust" collected in a vacuum cleaner is actually skin scales (squames) shed by people living in the house. They are also the major source of food for house dust mites, living in beds and soft furnishings.

The epidermis comprises primarily of living and dead keratinocytes. In addition, however, are other minority cell populations having specialised functions. This includes dendritic cells called "Langerhans cells" which comprise 2% of the total cell population. These are specialist cells of the immune system called antigen presenting cells. Their role is to detect and phagocytose foreign material that invades the skin, to digest and process the material, and to present epitopes of foreign antigens on its cell surface. It then migrates to lymph nodes where the foreign epitopes are presented to lymphocytes which can then mount an appropriate immunological response. Therefore, in addition to presenting physical barriers to invasion, skin also has immunological surveillance barriers.

9.1.2 Dermis

The dermis is the layer directly beneath the epidermis. The basement membrane separates the epidermis from the dermis. The dermis is a much thicker layer over 3mm thick. Unlike the epidermis which is comprised primarily of living and dead cells, the dermis is made up largely of extracellular matrix material particularly protein, within which the occasional cell is located. The cell largely responsible for manufacturing the extracellular matrix is the fibroblast cell. The dermal matrix also supports a number of specialist structures. This includes the vascular supply network including arteries, veins and capillaries. These supply nutrients and oxygen to all of the cells and other structures in the dermis. There are no blood vessels in the epidermis. The basal keratinocytes gain their supplies from capillaries just under the basement membrane in the dermis, by diffusion across the basement membrane.

Various nerve endings and receptors are also found in the dermis to detect heat, pain, touch etc.

At intervals, the epidermis descends down into the dermis to form a number of blind ending tubes. In this case the basement membrane and epidermis is located on the inside of the tube, and the dermis surrounds the tube. These structures include the hair follicles and sweat glands. These are the only cells of epithelial origin present in the depths of the dermis. They descend into the dermis to differing depths, so the deeper one goes the less epithelial appendages there will be. This has very important consequences for the wound healing process (see next section).

The extracellular matrix within the dermis gives skin its toughness and elasticity. The protein most responsible for toughness is collagen. Collagen is a fibrous protein, which is assembled into fibrils and the fibrils into fibres resembling the way in which rope is constructed. The fibres are orientated along the direction of greatest stress thus ensuring maximum strength. Collagen is the protein found in greatest quantity within the dermis. The next commonest structural protein in dermis is elastin. As the name suggests elastin is responsible for the elasticity of skin.

9.2   Wound Healing (Skin Regeneration)

How the body responds to a wound, and whether it is able to regenerate lost skin depends on many factors. One of the most important is the size of the wound (i.e. % of the body surface damaged) and the depth of the wound.

9.2.1   Epidermis-Only Wound

The most superficial type of wound is the epidermis-only wound. A good example of this would be sunburn. The damaged epidermis peels off but there is no bleeding (as there are no blood vessels in the epidermis). The epidermis is regenerated by faster proliferation of the basal keratinocytes. Once the stratum corneum is re-established the body is no longer at risk. Indeed, the old stratum corneum often does not peel away until a new one has formed underneath.

9.2.2   Partial Thickness Wound

A partial thickness wound comprises of damage to, or removal of, the epidermal layer and some of the dermis. This means that part of the body is no longer protected by an epithelial layer and the primary objective of the healing process is to restore this layer. Some of the re-epithelialisation takes place as a result of proliferation and migration of keratinocytes from the wound margins (edges). However, a second crucial source of keratinocytes is from the remnants of the epithelial appendages found in the wound bed (i.e. the remainders of the hair follicles and sweat glands).

In reality up to 90% of the new epithelium may derive from these wound bed remnants. However, the deeper the wound, the fewer remnants will be present, hence the longer the re-epithelialisation process will take. Once re-epithelialisation has been achieved the major risks to the body will have been averted. At the same time, the missing dermis matrix will be replaced by the rapid production of collagen by fibroblast cells. This is accompanied by angiogenesis, the formation of new blood vessels, to support this vigorous metabolic activity. The collagen is laid down in a random orientation to fill the void, as quickly as possible and an excess of blood vessels at this stage can result in a red raised scar. This will resolve through time.

9.2.3   Full Thickness Wound

A full thickness wound results in the removal or destruction of the whole skin thickness, such as a result of large severe burn injury. In this case the only source of epithelium to re-surface the wound is from the wound edges. For anything other than a tiny full thickness wound the time required for re-surfacing from the wound edges would be so slow that other processes such as wound infection or fibrosis, are likely to occur in the meantime thus preventing the re-epithelialisation process. Therefore, in reality, the only way to heal a full thickness wound is to use a split skin autograft. This comprises of taking a split skin graft from an area of undamaged skin and transferring this to the wound area (Figure 2). The skin graft very rapidly gains a blood supply as a result of blood vessels in the wound bed fusing with blood vessels in the graft, a process called "enosculation".

Obviously, by taking a skin graft, a second wound has been created. However, this is only a partial thickness injury so that the donor-site would be expected to heal in the same way that any other partial thickness injury would heal.

Although the use of split skin autografting revolutionised burn treatment, there can still be problems. Sometimes the grafts fail to attach or are destroyed by infection. Where the injury covers more than 50% of the body surface there is clearly insufficient undamaged skin left to provide enough grafts to cover the wound. Therefore, even with the advent of split skin autografting, the larger the burn the poorer the prognosis. Another major factor affecting the outcome of a large burn injury is the age of the patient with higher mortality in older patients. The figure below shows the mortality probability for a 50% body surface area burn for patients in different age groups (Figure 3).

Figure 2. Treatment of Full Thickness Wounds

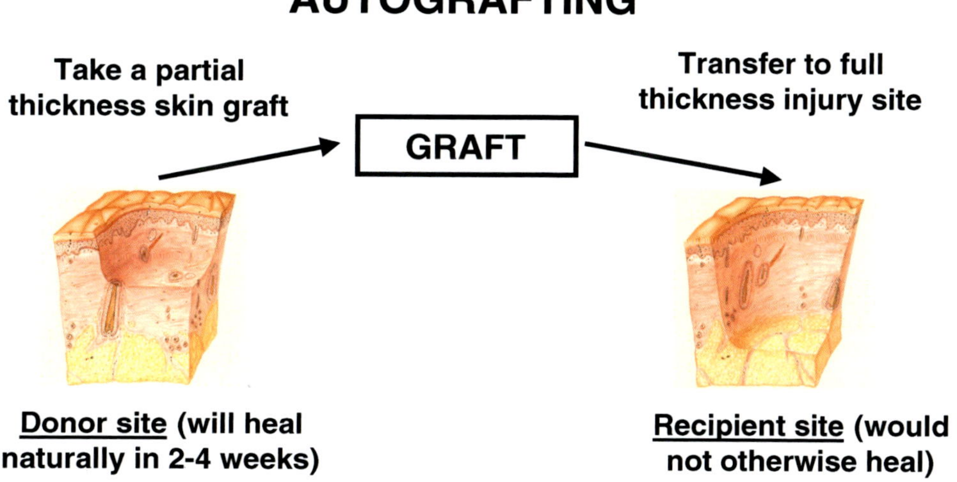

Figure 3. Morbidity after Burns and Age

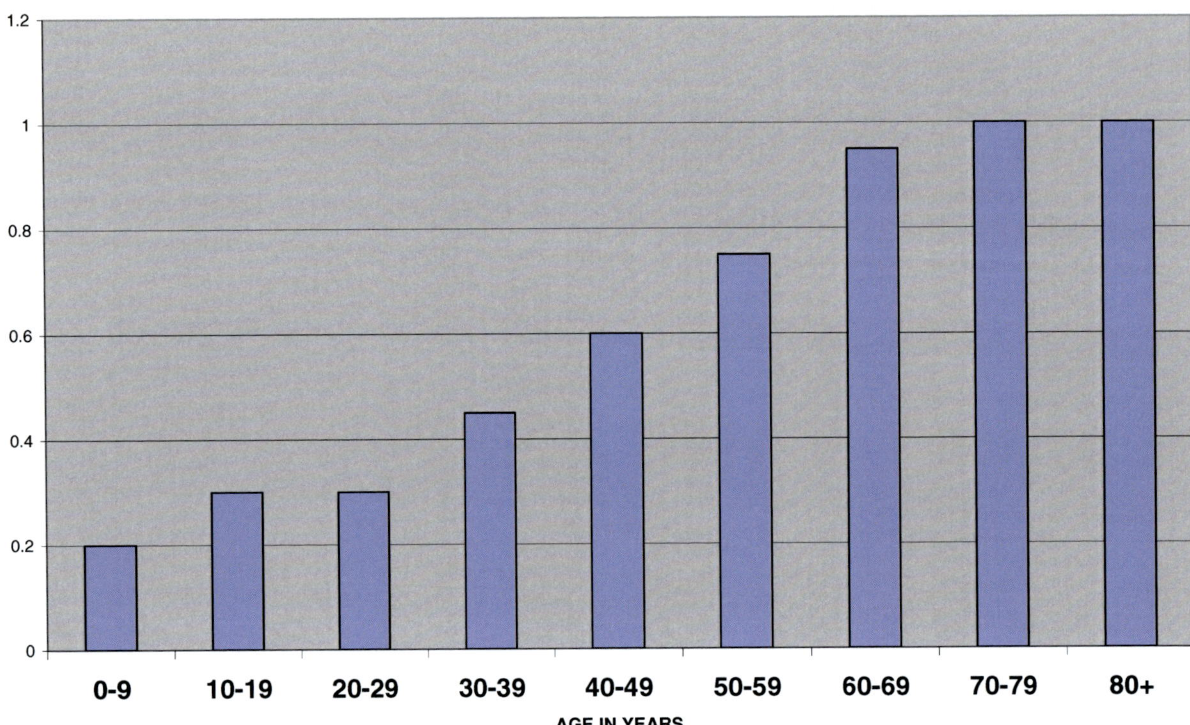

Adapted from Bull (1971) Lancet 2, 1133-1134

9.3   Use of Allografts

Skin allografts can be used where there are insufficient autografts to close the wound. Viable skin allografts (cryopreserved) will exhibit "graft take" and gain a blood supply in exactly the same way as an autograft. In contrast, non-viable (irradiated) skin allografts do not gain a blood supply and simply attach to the wound bed via fibrin which links collagen in the graft with collagen in the wound bed. It therefore acts as a biological dressing. Nevertheless, because the allograft has an intact stratum corneum it still provides a water-proofing, and bacteria-proofing function. After some days the weak bonds between graft and wound bed are broken down and the graft is sloughed off.

Whereas non-living allografts are removed passively, viable allografts are actively rejected. Skin tissue is highly immunogenic by virtue of its population of dendritic "Langerhans cells" of the immune system. In a normal immunocompetent recipient a skin graft will be rejected in 7-10 days. The recipients immune system attacks blood vessel cells in the graft which results in blockage of the capillaries and hence necrosis of the graft. Rejection can be avoided if the patient is given immunosuppressive drugs. However, these can make a burn patient more susceptible to infection, so are rarely given. However, one feature of very large burn wounds is that the patient becomes naturally immunosuppressed as a result of the effects of the injury on the immune system. Therefore viable skin allografts can survive for weeks or even months before being rejected. This "buys time" for the surgeon to use other methods. One example is that once the original autograft donor sites have healed, a second crop of grafts can be harvested. Alternatively the surgeon may use the time to apply tissue engineering skin culture methods to grow some of the patient's epithelium in vitro. Therefore, even though the viable skin allografts are ultimately rejected, they can prove to be critical, life-saving grafts.

9.4   Suggested Reading

1. Kearney J. Banking of skin grafts and biological dressings. In: *Principles and Practice of Burns Management*. (Ed. John A D Settle). Churchill Livingstone. 329-351 (1996).

2. Kearney JN. et al. Cryopreservation of skin using a murine model: validation of a prognostic viability assay. Cryobiology, 27:23-30 (1990).

3. Kearney JN. et al. Effects of cryobiological variables on the survival of skin using a defined murine model. Cryobiology, 27:164-170 (1990).

4. Ingham E. et al. The effects of variation of cryopreservation protocols on the immunogenicity of allogeneic skin grafts. Cryobiology, 30:443-458 (1993).

5. Kearney JN. Wound Healing. In: *Principles and Practice of Burns Management*. (Ed. John A D Settle) Churchill Livingstone. 187-195 (1996).

6. Kearney JN. Quality issues in skin banking: a review. Burns, 24:299-305 (1998).

7. Kearney JN. Clinical evaluation of skin substitutes. Burns 27:545-551 (2001).

8. Huang Q. et al. Use of peracetic acid to sterilise human donor skin for production of acellular dermal matrices for clinical use. Wound Repair and Regeneration.12:276-287 (2004).

9. Kearney JN. Guidelines on processing and clinical use of skin allografts. Clinics in Dermatology 23:357-364 (2005).

9.5   Self Assessment Questions

Multiple Choice Questions
1. Which of the following are true? The epidermis …
    a) Comprises 98% fibroblasts
    b) Comprises 98% Langerhans cell
    c) Comprises 98% keratinocytes
    d) Is 0.05 to 0.15 mm thick
    e) Is 0.5 to 1.5 mm thick

2. Which of the following are true of burn injuries?
    a) Mortality increases with increasing size of wound
    b) Mortality decreases with increasing size of wound
    c) Mortality increases with patient age
    d) Mortality decreases with patient age
    e) Mortality is not related to patient age

3. Which of the following are true?
    a) The epidermis and dermis are of equal thickness
    b) The epidermis is thicker than the dermis
    c) The dermis is thicker than the epidermis
    d) Squames are found in the epidermis
    e) Squames are found in the dermis

4. Which of the following are true?
    a) The basal layer is found in the dermis
    b) The stratum corneum is next to the basal layer
    c) The stratum corneum is the outermost layer of the dermis
    d) The stratum corneum is the outermost layer of the epidermis
    e) Stem cells are found in the stratum corneum

Short Answer Questions
1. What are the advantages and disadvantages of using living skin allografts?
2. What is split skin autografting?

Assignments
1. Compare and contrast the performance of alternative skin substitutes.
2. Why do large full thickness burn injuries not heal naturally without the need for skin grafts?

10 BIOLOGY OF MUSCULO-SKELETAL TISSUE

The human leg consists of the thigh and the lower leg. It contains four bones - femur (thigh), patella (kneecap), tibia (lower leg) and fibula (lower leg) as well as a number of muscles and ligaments (Figure 1). The leg contains one major synovial joint – the knee with the hip and ankle joints at either end of the leg.

Figure 1. Bones of the Leg.

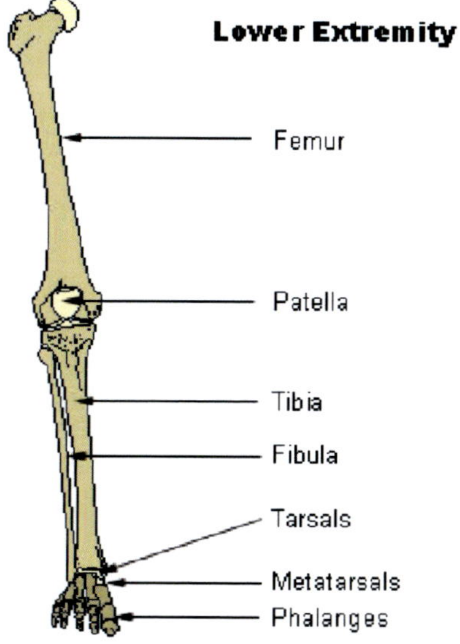

10.1 Overview of Bone

Bone is a rigid tissue that forms part of the endoskeleton of vertebrates. There are five types of bone in the body - long bones, flat bones, short bones, irregular bones and sesamoid bones that all form in one of two ways – by "endochondral ossification" or by "intramembraneous ossification". Endochondral ossification is the main form of bone formation and bones form by first making a cartilage model and includes all of the long bones of the body whereas intramembraneous bones form by mesenchymal cells differentiating directly into bone and include bones such as the flat bones of the skull. The leg contains long bones (femur, tibia, fibula) and a sesamoid bone (patella) which forms within a tendon.

Bone has five main functions: support, protection, movement, haematopoiesis and mineral storage. Some also have specialised functions such as ear bones aiding hearing or the storage of triglycerides and other bioactive molecules. The function of a mature bone is not dependent on the way it forms.

10.2 Long Bone Formation and Bone Growth - Endochondral Ossification.

Mesenchymal cells migrate to the site of the eventual bone formation and the cells differentiate into chondrocytes - at this stage the chondrocytes are rounded or spherical in shape. The chondrocytes secrete extracellular matrix and the cells separate to form the shape of the presumptive bone (Figure 2). The outer cells of the cartilage model become stretched and form a perichondrium which surrounds the tissue and the chondrocytes take on three distinct morphologies – some stay rounded with high cell proliferation potential, some become flattened along the short axis to resemble a coin and some swell and become hypertrophic. The three types of chondrocyte are arranged in five zones along the length of the rudiment – rounded, flattened, hypertrophic, flattened, rounded. In humans, cartilage long bone rudiments of the arms and legs form by the eighth week of foetal life.

Figure 2. Diagrammatic Representation of Bone Formation

[From Sadava et al. The Science of Biology. Used with Permission.]

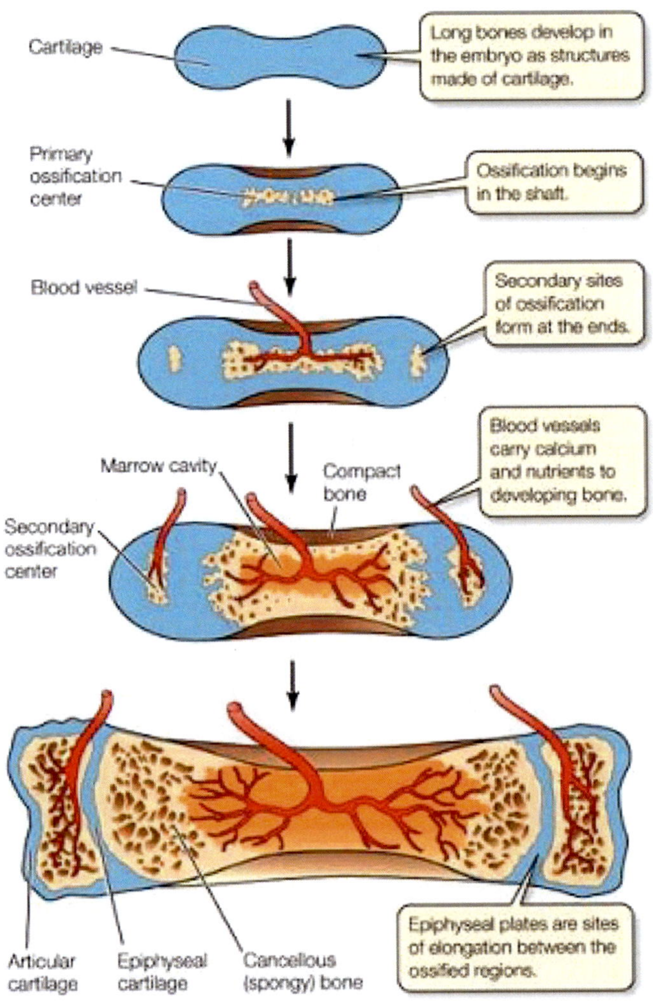

Around the ninth week blood vessels migrate into the centre of the hypertrophic zone from the perichondrium and the hypertrophic cells die (Figure 2). Other cells migrate in with blood vessels, some of these erode and remove the chondrocytes and mesenchymal stem cells differentiate into osteoblasts which attach to the extracellular matrix and lay down a specialised matrix called osteoid which subsequently mineralises - this site is called the primary ossification centre.

When the osteoblasts lay down sufficient mineral, they become trapped, can no longer divide and become osteocytes. The surrounding perichondrium also changes and becomes a fibrous periosteum and cells within the periosteum also differentiate into osteoblasts and then osteocytes. Not all of the central region becomes bone, there are still regions of blood vessels and connective tissue and these regions form the bone marrow cavity embedded within trabeculae of cancellous bone. Towards the periosteum, gaps between trabeculae get filled in to form a solid bony structure - called cortical bone (Figures 2 and 3).

As ossification proceeds within the centre of the long bone rudiment, flattened chondrocytes become hypertrophic and these too are resorbed and replaced by bone. In this way, ossification moves from the centre towards the ends. Secondary ossification centres form within the rounded chondrocyte zones leaving a portion of cartilage at the extremities which becomes articular cartilage and a portion below the secondary centre which becomes the epiphyseal growth plate (Figure 2). All future growth in length of the bone occurs through cell division, extracellular matrix secretion and hypertrophy by chondrocytes in the growth plate followed by erosion and replacement by bone.

Figure 3. Transverse Section through a Femur Showing Dense Cortical Bone on the Outside with Bone Marrow and Cancellous Bone in the Interior.

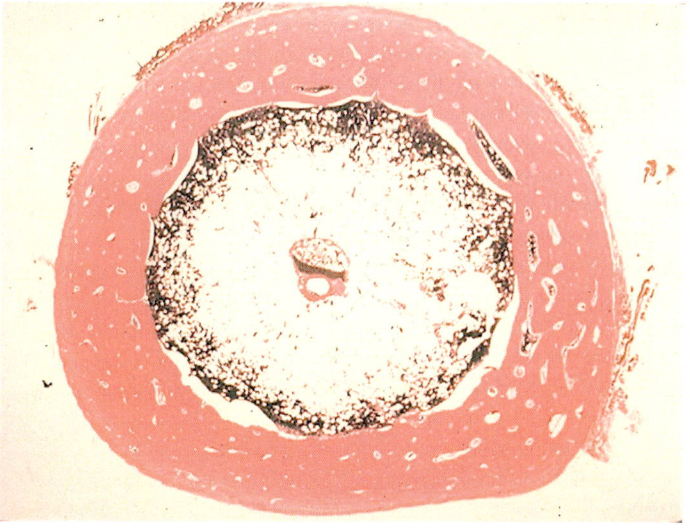

When skeletal maturity is reached, the chondrocytes in the growth place undergo hypertrophy, become eroded and replaced by bone, the epiphysis is "closed", it fuses with the rest of the bone and growth in length ceases. Bone is not a fixed, permanent structure, it continues to change shape and remodel on a microscopic scale due to dynamic forces, normal wear and tear and as a result of fracture. Bone tissue is eroded by osteoclasts which are multinucleated cells derived from the monocyte/macrophage lineage.

10.3 Bone Characteristics

By its nature, cancellous bone is composed of bony trabeculae within a more open bone marrow structure and is therefore relatively lightweight but still hard. Cortical bone does not have gaps between layers (Figure 3). The mineral is mostly calcium phosphate in the form of hydroxyapatite. Bone has relatively high compressive strength but poor tensile strength, i.e. it resists pushing forces well but not pulling forces. A long bone is generally composed of approximately 80% cortical bone and 20% cancellous bone by weight, although, due to its trabecular nature, cancellous bone has nearly 10 times the surface area of cortical bone.

10.4 Bone Functions

Support – The skeleton provides a rigid internal framework for the body. It supports all the internal organs and provides a point for muscle and tendon/ligament attachment.

Protection – The skeleton protects internal organs from injury: the cranium protects the brain; vertebrae protect the spinal cord; rib cage protects the heart and lungs.

Movement – Bones, skeletal muscles, tendons, ligaments and joints function together to generate and transfer forces so that individual body parts or the whole body can be manipulated in three-directions.

Haematopoiesis – Red blood cells, white blood cells and platelets are all made within red bone marrow located in the epiphyses of longs bones, ribs, sternum, skull bones and bony vertebral bodies. In young children all bone marrow is red bone marrow but as they grow older most red marrow converts to yellow marrow which is primarily involved with triglyceride storage.

Mineral storage – Bone acts as a reservoir for storage of calcium and phosphorous which are released as ions to participate in various physiological reactions throughout the body. Calcium ions released from bone matrix are used in muscle contraction. Various hormones acting on osteoblasts and osteoclasts control the storage and release of the ions.

10.5 Bone Remodelling.

Remodelling is the process of bone resorption, by osteoclasts, followed by laying down new bone by osteoblasts - this causes little change in shape and occurs throughout life. Its purpose is the release of calcium and the repair of micro-damage. Repeated stress results in the bone thickening at the points of maximum stress.

Osteoblasts (Figure 4) are bone-forming cells, derived from mesenchymal stem cells. They synthesise and secrete extracellular matrix, osteoid, which mineralises. The cells are capable of cell division until late stages when they become trapped in mineralised matrix and become osteocytes.

Osteocytes are fully differentiated bone cells, derived from trapped osteoblasts. They are located within lacunae and communicate with other cells via long processes known as cannaniculi.

Osteoclasts are the cells responsible for bone resorption. They are large, multinucleated cells, produce enzymes which breakdown old bone by producing "resorption pits" which osteoblasts then migrate into to lay down new bone.

Figure 4. Histological Section of Bone Showing the Major Bone Cell Types

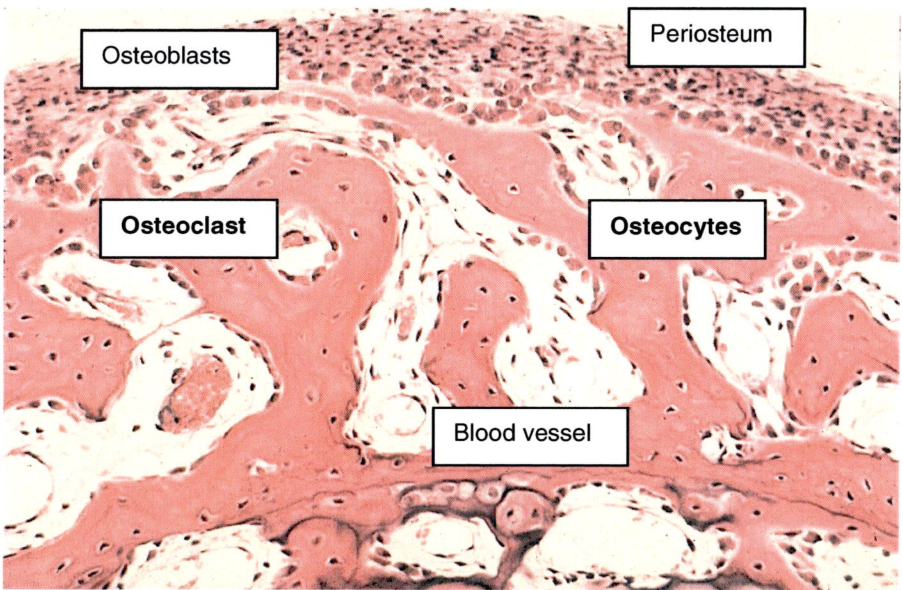

10.6 The Knee Joint.

The knee joint comprises the distal femur and proximal tibia separated by the meniscus but held together by the patella tendon and cruciate ligaments (Figure 5).

Figure 5. Diagrammatic Representation of a Knee Joint

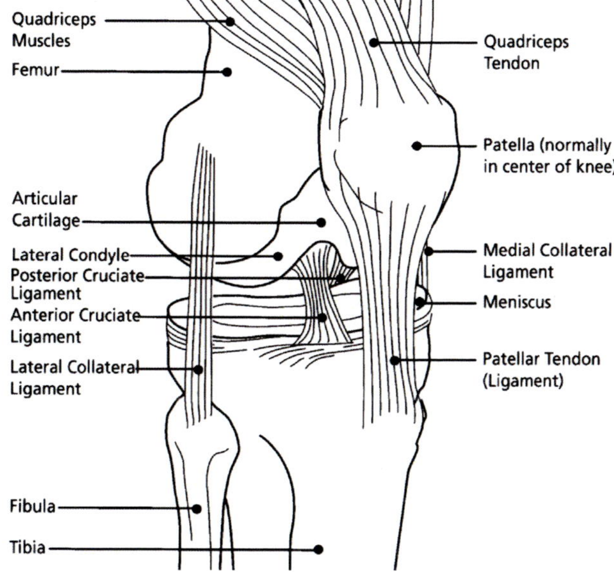

Tendons join skeletal muscle to bone, they are often long and straight but can also be very short. They transmit force in one direction and act as shock absorbers. They sometimes pass through a groove or sheath and can be stretched 5 - 10% before injury. A tendon can absorb more strain energy per unit weight than any other tissue.

Ligaments join bone to bone, they are often short but can also be fat/irregular sheets. These tissues often resist forces in more than one direction and play a role as major shock absorbers.

The knee joint contains two sections of meniscus - the lateral meniscus and the medial meniscus. Both are cartilaginous tissues that provide structural integrity to the knee when it undergoes tension and torsion. Both menisci are half-moon "C" shapes, which disperse friction between the tibia and the femur during movement and spread the load of a body's weight.

10.7 Suggested Reading

Alberts B. et al. Histology: the lives and deaths of cells in tissues. In, *Molecular Biology of the Cell.* 4th edn. Chapter 22.

Board TN. et al. Impaction allografting in revision total hip replacement. J. Bone Jt. Surg. 88B: 852-857 (2006).

Cancedda R. et al. Bone marrow stromal cells and their use in regenerating bone. In, *Tissue Engineering of Cartilage and Bone.* Eds. G. Beck and J. Goode, Novartis Foundation Symposium 248. Pp 133-143 (2003).

Dellloye C et al. *Impaction bone grafting in revision arthroplasty.* Marcel Dekker Inc New York. (2004).

Hofer S. et al. Clinical perspectives of the use of bone grafts based on allografts. In, *Bone Graft Substitutes.* Ed. CT Laurencin. Pp 68 - 95 (2003).

Joyce MJ et al. Musculoskeletal allograft tissue banking and safety. In, *Bone Graft Substitutes.* Ed. CT Laurencin. Pp 30 -58 (2003).

Kaur C. Histology of bone. In, *The Scientific Basis of Tissue Transplantation, Advances in Tissue Banking vol. 5.* Ed. A. Nather. World Scientific Publishing. Pp 97 - 114 (2001).

Kearney JN et al. The osteoinductive properties of demineralised bone matrix. In, *Advances in Tissue Banking Vol. 1.* Eds. GO Phillips, R von Versen, DM Strong, A Nather. World Scientific Publishing. Pp 43 - 71 (1997).

Nather A. Anatomy of the lower limb. In, *The Scientific Basis of Tissue Transplantation, Advances in Tissue Banking Vol. 5.* Ed. A. Nather. World Scientific Publishing. Pp 25 - 41 (2001).

10.8 Self Assessment Questions

Multiple Choice Questions

1. How many different types of bone are there?
    a) 1
    b) 2
    c) 3
    d) 4
    e) 5

2. What two cell types are involved in bone remodelling?
    a) Osteoblasts and osteocytes
    b) Osteocytes and osteoclasts
    c) Osteoblasts and osteoclasts
    d) Osteoblasts and chondrocytes
    e) Osteocytes only

3. A tendon joins skeletal muscle to what?
    a) Another tendon
    b) Bone
    c) Ligaments
    d) Cartilage
    e) Smooth muscle

4. What is the main type of bone formation in the leg?
    a) Intramembraneous ossification
    b) New bone formation
    c) Endochochondral ossification
    d) Fracture repair
    e) Osteocytosis

Short Answer Questions

1. List the five main functions of bone.
2. What does the term "endochondral ossification" mean and how is it different from intramembraneous ossification?

Assignments

1. How are different musculoskeletal tissues processed and why are they processed differently?
2. Surgeons do not always use allograft bone during bone repair or transplantation - what other bone substitutes are available and why may they be preferred?

11 BIOLOGY OF CARDIOVASCULAR TISSUE

Several cardiovascular tissues are banked for use as tissue grafts. These can be categorised into heart valves, pericardium and blood vessels. Note that hyperlinks to relevant diagrams and photographs are given at the end of this chapter.

11.1 Heart Valves

There are four valves located within the heart. The tricuspid and mitral (or bicuspid) valves separate the right atrium and ventricle and the left atrium and ventricle respectively, the aortic valve separates the left ventricle and aorta, and the pulmonary valve separates the right ventricle and the trunk of the pulmonary artery.

The function of the valves is to divide different parts of the heart and the major blood vessels leaving the heart, and to permit blood to flow in only one direction. This is accomplished by the cusps (or leaflets) within the valve. The pulmonary valve and the aortic valve are sometimes termed semi-lunar valves because both contain three half-moon (semi-lunar) shaped leaflets.

Problems with heart valves can be either congenital or acquired. Congenital defects include transposition of the great arteries where the pulmonary artery leads off the left ventricle and the aorta off the right ventricle, tetralogy of Fallot and congenital pulmonary stenosis. Most of these conditions are accompanied by atrial or ventral septal defects (holes in the heart) between the two atria to ventricles and transposition would be fatal if there was not a septal defect as there would be two closed circulations, one to lungs and one to body. Heart valves can become damaged or diseased due to a number of factors like bacterial or viral infections, lifestyle factors, such as poor diet or smoking, or simply due to ageing. This damage can take two basic forms; either the valve becomes too narrow (stenosis) which restricts blood flow through the valve, or they fail to close properly, allowing blood to be regurgitated the wrong way through the valve. Left untreated, this can result in heart failure so it is therefore important that when a valve begins to fail it is repaired or replaced.

Cardiac surgeons have a number of options available to replace damaged valves. These comprise prosthetic grafts, bioprosthetic grafts, allografts or autografts. The majority of heart valve replacement operations utilise prosthetic or bioprosthetic grafts. Fully prosthetic valves are entirely synthetic being made from pyrolytic carbon in titanium stent covered with Dacron. Bioprosthetic valves are formed by suturing a porcine valve either into a Dacron covered metal stent or into a Dacron tube. The porcine tissue has been treated with glutaraldehyde which crosslinks, strengthens and sterilises the tissue. In a cardiac autograft operation (also termed a Ross Procedure) the surgeon places the patient's pulmonary valve in the aortic position and then an allograft in the pulmonary position.

Heart valve allografts can be obtained from donors up to the age of 65 with most banks using 6 months as lower age limit. Nowadays the only   heart valves used for allograft are pulmonary or aortic valves, but in the past mitral valves were also used. Almost all valves are obtained from deceased donors, although there are occasions where a living person undergoing a heart transplant can donate valves from their original heart. Paediatric heart valve allografts have always been in short supply as in this age group allografts are used in preference to prosthetic and bioprosthetic valves. Usually when taken for tissue donation, the entire heart is removed and returned to the tissue bank, as it is not practical to dissect out individual valves at the site of donation. It is preferable when retrieving a heart for valve donation to remove as much of the blood vessels associated with the valves (the aorta and pulmonary artery), as a longer vessel length increases the utility of the valves to surgeons.

Different banking methodologies have been used for heart valves, however all heart valve banks in Europe today disinfect the graft with antibiotics and then cryopreserve it. There has been a long-standing debate about the importance of donor cell viability in heart valve allografts. It was previously thought that this was important as donor cells would help maintain and repair the valve tissue. However, studies have shown that donor cells very rapidly disappear from the graft after implantation. The balance of current opinion suggests that the presence of viable donor cells may actually be a disadvantage, as they can lead to an increased immunogenic response against the graft.

Following donation, the heart is returned to the tissue bank on wet ice wrapped in moist antiseptic gauze, to prevent moisture loss and reduce surface contamination. The pulmonary and aortic valves are then dissected out (Figure 1) and carefully examined. The anatomical structure of the valves is looked at to ensure that no cuts, holes or other anatomical abnormalities are present. The valves are then partially inverted to look for the presence of atherosclerosis (yellow, fatty deposits), calcification (hard, mineral deposits) and fenestrations (natural holes in the cusps normally where they would meet when valve closes) on the valve leaflets and blood vessel walls. The presence of this type of pathology indicates that the valve will be more prone to deteriorate following implantation, and calcification and atheroma is common in valves from older donors.

Figure 1. Dissected Aortic Heart Valve

Note the coronary arteries, which have been sutured off at the base of the aorta.

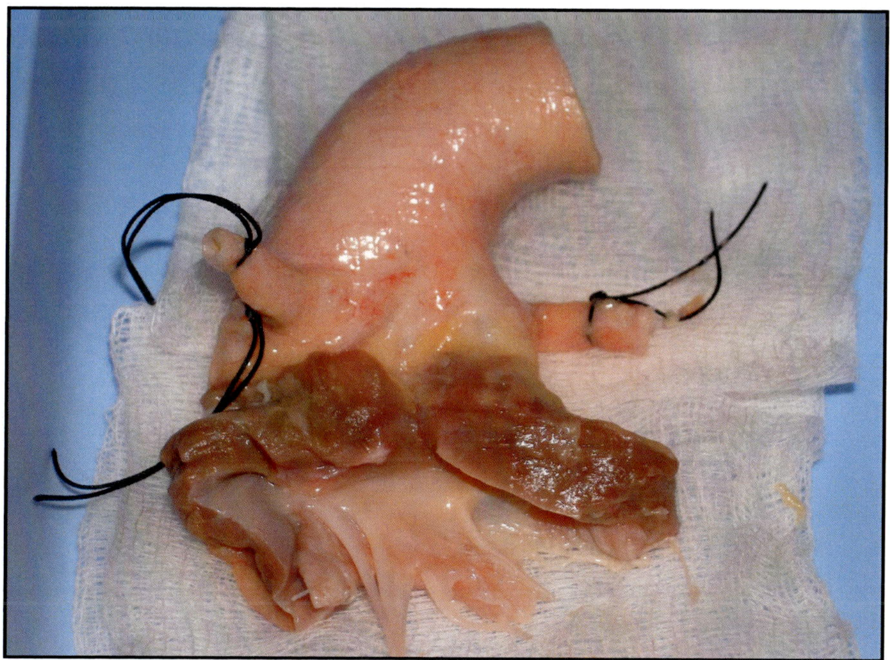

In addition to the pathology of the valve, its competency must also be assessed. The term competency refers to ability of the valve to hold fluid, and prevent it leaking, which would indicate that it may cause regurgitation. To assess competency, the valve is held in its normal configuration and filled with a physiological solution. The annular diameter of the valve is measured as this needs to be closely matched to that of the recipient at time of implantation. This is determined using blunt ended obturators. Some banks will re-measure the valve after dissection as it has been known for valves to shrink during this process. The length of the blood vessels is also recorded.

Following dissection and assessment of pathology, the valves are decontaminated by immersion in antibiotic solution.

The need to avoid damage to the tissue structure and to preserve tissue viability means that this is the only decontamination that can be applied. As the antibiotics used can bind to the tissue, it is possible that assessing the microbial status of the graft after decontamination may result in false negative results. For this reason, the microbial status of the valve both before and after decontamination is assessed. The valves are then packaged, and cryopreserved for long term storage.

11.2 Pericardium

The pericardium is a fibrous membrane that completely surrounds the heart, enclosing it in a sac. It does not directly join to the heart muscle, but secretes a thin layer of fluid that separates it from the heart. It has three main functions:

- It prevents the heart from over-expanding when it beats
- It is joined to the diaphragm, and secures the heart in position within the chest cavity
- The thin fluid layer protects the heart from friction when it beats

As the pericardium completely surrounds the heart, any open cardiac surgery requires that the pericardium be opened. When this has been done, the incision in the pericardium cannot be sutured, but has to be replaced with a patch, secured to either side of the incision. As with heart valves, there are different grafting options available to surgeons. Prosthetic Dacron patches, or patches made from processed and cross linked bovine pericardium are available. However, these materials integrate very poorly with native pericardium, and for this reason pericardium allografts are also in demand. It is thought that acellular pericardium allograft will be even more suitable for this purpose, as the absence of donor cells will accelerate the rate at which the recipient's cells could repopulate the graft. Pericardium has also been used for patching atrial and septal defects and for producing conduits particularly in congenital cardiac surgery.

11.3 Blood Vessels

Arteries and veins form the major part of the circulatory system, with arteries transporting oxygenated blood from the heart to the body's organs and tissues, and veins returning de-oxygenated blood to the heart. As with heart valves, blood vessels are subject to vascular disease, for very much the same reasons. Dietary and lifestyle factors result in vascular disease being very common in middle aged and elderly patients. Vascular disease affecting larger arteries and veins begins with the deposition of atherosclerotic plaques of fatty material on the inner walls of blood vessels. These plaques gradually increase in size with the deposition of ever more fatty material, until the blood vessel becomes very narrow or is blocked entirely. Occasionally, these plaques can break away from vessel wall and block smaller bore vessels elsewhere in the body. Arterial walls can also thin with age or disease and then bulge to form aneurysms which can eventually rupture and haemorrhage.

If coronary arteries (the arteries which supply the heart muscle with blood) become blocked, a heart attack results. Even with larger arteries, which are less likely to be fully blocked, the build up of atherosclerosis is associated with increasing calcification of the vessel wall. This makes the vessel less flexible and weaker, so more prone to rupture which has a high mortality rate when occurring in thoracic or abdominal arteries.

Options for replacement of blocked or damaged blood vessels include prosthetic graft, autograft and allograft. A commonly used and very successful autografting procedure involves using a section of saphenous vein or internal mammary artery to form a bypass graft, circumventing the blocked artery.

For damaged larger arteries, the treatment of choice is usually prosthetic grafts, such as the Dacron prosthesis shown below. Here, the femoral artery has developed a severe aneurysm, and the weakened section of artery needs to be replaced. The Dacron graft is spliced into position after removal of the artery.

However, in some cases, prosthetic grafts can become very badly infected. In these situations, replacement with another prosthetic graft is not desirable, as it would be likely to become infected also. In these situations, surgeons prefer to use artery allografts as these are more resistant to infection. In this situation, the artery graft (Figure 2) is a treatment of last resort.

Figure 2. Artery Allografts (Thoracic Aorta and Aorto-Illiac Grafts)

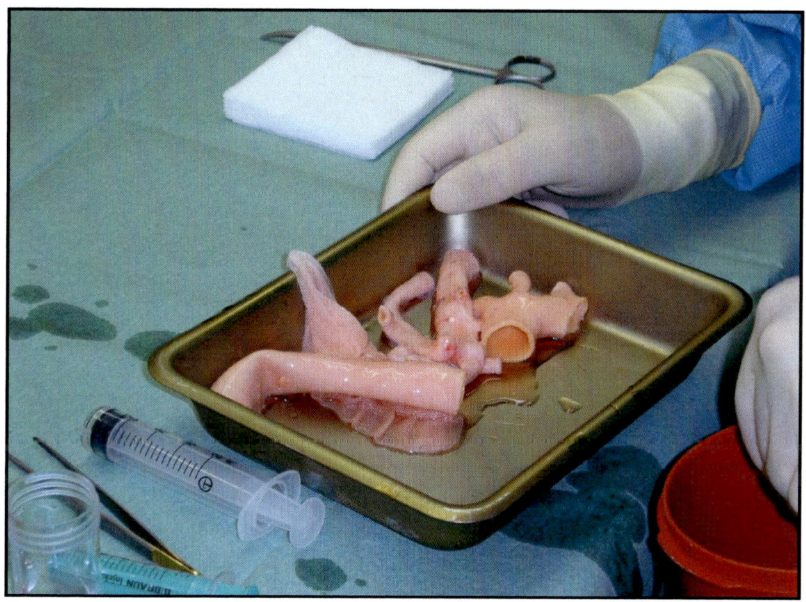

11.4 Suggested Reading

Good web site on prosthetic heart valves:
http://cape.uwaterloo.ca/che100projects/heart/files/testing.htm

Leeming JP. et al. Residual antibiotics in allograft heart valve tissue samples following antibiotic disinfection. Hosp Infect. 60:231-234 (2005).

Dexter F. et al. Post-mortem shrinkage of homograft aortic valves. Thorax 27:312-314 (1972).

Mirsadraee S. et al. Development and characterization of an acellular human pericardial matrix for tissue engineering. Tissue Eng. 12:763-773 (2006).

Yankah AC et al. *Cardiac Valve Allografts II: Science and Practice*. Darmstadt. (1996).

Hopkins RA. *Cardiac Reconstruction with Allograft Tissue*. Springer-Verlag. (2004).

Other Web-Based Diagrams and Photographs

The anatomical location of heart valves and their relationship to blood flow:
http://www.internet-encyclopedia.org/upload/1/15/Heart_labelled_large.png

Prosthetic and bioprosthetic heart valves:
http://cape.uwaterloo.ca/che100projects/heart/files/testing.htm

The pericardium and its relationship to the heart:
http://health.yahoo.com/topic/heart/overview/article/healthwise/popup/tp10894

Formation of atherosclerotic plaques:
http://www.surrey.ac.uk/SBMS/MicrobialSciences/research/immunology.htm

Coronary artery bypass grafting procedure:
http://www.ohioheartandvascular.com/cvprocedures/coronary-bypass-surgery.php

Aneurysm using a Dacron graft:
http://www.jvascbr.com.br/03-02-02/03-02-02-145/03-02-02-145.htm

11.5 Self Assessment Questions

Multiple Choice Questions

1. Heart valves from which animal are used to make bioprosthetic valves?
   a) Pigs
   b) Chimpanzees
   c) Cows
   d) Sheep
   e) Rats

2. Which of the following lifestyle factors does NOT damage heart valves?
   a) Poor diet
   b) Smoking
   c) Old age
   d) Regular exercise
   e) Pregnancy

3. What term is used to describe fatty deposits on the surface of heart valves?
   a) Atherosclerosis
   b) Lipidoma
   c) Calcification
   d) Arteriolosclerosis
   e) Arteriosclerosis

4. What substance can be used to make prosthetic artery and pericardium grafts?
   a) Teflon
   b) Dacron
   c) Nylon
   d) Rayon
   e) Polypropylene

Short Answer Questions

1. Which two chambers in the heart are separated by the mitral valve?
2. Why might the presence of viable cells in a heart valve graft be undesirable?

Assignments

1. Discuss the advantages and disadvantages of prosthetic and bioprosthetic grafts in relation to allografts.
2. How can a graft be decellularised? What are the risks of decellularising a graft, in terms of damage to its biological and biomechanical properties?

12 BIOLOGY OF OCULAR TISSUE

12.1 Background

Corneal transplantation is the oldest and most widely used forms of allographic solid tissue transplantation. Attempts at transplanting corneas were made in the early 1800s, with a successful graft on a pet gazelle being reported by Samuel Biggar in 1837. However, it was not until 1905 that the first successful full-thickness corneal transplant was achieved in a human by Eduard Zirm. The tissue for these early grafts came from living donors who had undergone therapeutic enucleation (removal of the eye) owing to ocular injuries or disease. In the 1930s, Filatov pioneered the use of corneas from deceased donors as well as the storage of whole eyes in closed pots (moist chambers) on ice. With the discovery of antibiotics and steroids, improvements in surgical instruments, suture materials, and introduction of operating microscopes, corneal transplantation became increasingly successful and widespread. Now, approximately 2500 corneal transplants are carried out every year in the UK compared with more than 30,000 p.a. in the USA.

12.2 Structure and Function of the Cornea

The cornea is the transparent foremost part of the eye. At the limbus, the transparent cornea merges into the white, opaque sclera. Together with the sclera, the cornea forms part of the tough outer coat of the eye and is an important barrier protecting the inner structures of the eye against infection and trauma. In humans the cornea is a little over 0.5 mm thick in the centre, becoming thicker towards the periphery, with a diameter of approximately 12 mm and a radius of curvature of about 8 mm. Its shape and remarkable transparency, with 85-95% of incident light in the visible spectrum being transmitted, mean that the cornea is a major refractive component of the eye. Because of its smooth outer (in part owing to the tear film) and inner surfaces and spherical shape, the cornea acts as a lens contributing about 70% of the total dioptric (focussing) power of the eye. By contrast, the crystalline lens behind the pupil contributes only 30% of dioptric power but is important for accommodation, the ability to focus images at both near and far distances. It is the crystalline lens that becomes cloudy through the development of cataracts and is replaced by an artificial intraocular lens during cataract surgery.

A transverse section through cornea reveals five distinct layers: an outer stratified epithelium, Bowman's layer, the stroma, Descemet's membrane and a monolayer of endothelium.

12.2.1 Epithelium

The epithelium is 5-7 cell layers thick. The basal columnar cells are transient amplifying cells that contribute to maintenance of the epithelial mass. As these basal cells divide, the daughter cells move towards the surface of the epithelium and the centre of the cornea becoming progressively more differentiated first into wing cells in the mid epithelium and then ending up as highly flattened superficial cells. These cells are interconnected by tight junctions and are responsible for the barrier properties of the epithelium. As they die, these superficial cells are shed of and continuously replaced by cells moving up from the lower epithelial layers. A population of epithelial stem cells residing at the limbus is thought to be the source of the transient amplifying cells. The epithelium is highly innervated and not only acts as a barrier to microbial organisms but is important for maintaining a healthy tear film. Ocular surface disease resulting from failure of the epithelium is difficult to treat and often has a poor prognosis. The epithelium has a basement membrane that sits on Bowman's layer, which is a non-cellular, modified region of the anterior stroma.

The epithelium also contains some antigen presenting cells, Langerhans cells, and these are typically confined to the peripheral one third of the cornea.

12.2.2 Stroma

The stroma forms 90% of the thickness of the cornea and its structure is critical to corneal transparency. The stroma is made up of parallel bundles of collagen fibrils embedded in proteoglycans. The fibrils are organized into sheets (lamellae) that lie parallel to each other. Keratocytes are specialized cells lying between the lamellae, and they synthesise collagen and proteoglycans. The diameter of the fibrils and the interfibrillar spacing are very uniform and it is this regular arrangement of the collagen fibrils that is responsible for the high degree of light transmission through the cornea. Disruption of this regular pattern, for example by stromal oedema, causes loss of transparency. There are also a few dendritic cells scattered throughout the stroma. The posterior stroma lies against Descemet's membrane, which is secreted by the endothelial cells and acts as their basement membrane. Abnormal stroma is a major reason for corneal transplantation, especially in keratoconus, a disease where the stroma becomes progressively thinner. The cornea also loses its spherical shape, becoming more conical and causing severe distortion of vision.

12.2.3 Endothelium

The endothelium is a monolayer of closely apposed, hexagonal cells, approximately 20 μm wide and 5 μm high. These cells are responsible for controlling stromal hydration, keeping the cornea thin and clear. Because the cornea is avascular, the keratocytes and epithelium rely on nutrients diffusing into the cornea across the endothelium from the aqueous humour. This influx is driven by the fixed negative charge of the stroma, which brings in ions and water. Failure to counter this influx of water would lead to stromal oedema and loss of transparency. The endothelium actively transports ions, including bicarbonate, from the stroma, which creates an osmotic gradient across the endothelium that balances the forces driving the water influx. This is an active metabolic process, which can be demonstrated by cooling cornea to inhibit the endothelial pump, which in turn causes stromal swelling and cloudiness. Warming the corneas to physiological temperature restores the endothelial pump and the corneas return to normal thickness. Another major indication for corneal transplantation is failure of the endothelium to maintain corneal transparency. This either comes about through specific corneal dystrophies or as a result of previous intraocular surgery, including cataract surgery, that can have a long-term damaging effect on the endothelium. The problem with human corneal endothelial cells is that they only a limited capacity for replication. Cell loss or damage is repaired by neighbouring cells migrating and spreading to fill gaps on Descemet's membrane. As a result, there is a gradual loss of endothelial cells throughout life and a decline in endothelial cell density.

12.3 Suggested Reading

Armitage WJ. et al. The first successful full-thickness corneal transplant: a commentary on Eduard Zirm's landmark paper of 1906. Br J Ophthalmol. 90:1222-1223 (2006).

Armitage WJ. et al. Factors influencing the suitability of organ-cultured corneas for transplantation. Invest Ophthalmol Vis Sci. 38:16-24 (1997)

Armitage WJ. et al. Predicting endothelial cell loss and long-term corneal graft survival. Invest Ophthalmol Vis Sci. 44:3326-3331 (2003).

Fuller BJ. et al. *Clinical Applications of Cryobiology*, CRC Press (1991).

Jeng BH. Preserving the cornea: corneal storage media. Curr Opinion Ophthalmol. 17:332-337 (2006).

Klyce SD. et al. Structure and function of the cornea. In, *The Cornea*. Eds HE Kaufman, BA Barron, MB McDonald. Butterworth-Heinemann (1998).

Pels E et al. Organ culture preservation of human corneas. Doc Ophthalmol. 56:147-153 (1983).

12.4 Self Assessment Questions

Multiple Choice Questions

1. What percentage of corneal thickness is taken up by the stroma?
   a) 75%
   b) 95%
   c) 80%
   d) 90%
   e) 10%

2. Which are the main resident cells in the corneal stroma?
   a) Keratinocytes
   b) Dendritic cells
   c) Keratocytes
   d) Langerhans
   e) Osteocytes

Short Answer Questions

1. Why are some malignancies in donors a contraindication to all tissue transplantation apart from cornea? What ocular tissues cannot be transplanted from these donors?

Assignments

1. Describe the role of the corneal endothelium and why it is critical to the success of the majority of corneal transplants.

STEM CELL TRANSPLANTATION SCIENCE

13 HAEMATOPOIETIC STEM CELL TRANSPLANTATION: AN OVERVIEW

13.1 What is Haematopoiesis?

Haematopoiesis refers to the production of blood and bone marrow cells. Haematopoietic stem cells (HSC), which are located in very small numbers within the bone marrow, give rise to all the cells of the haematopoietic system. These cells divide asymmetrically so that a division results in another stem cell (to maintain the stocks of haematopoietic progenitor cell (HPCs)) and a slightly more differentiated HPC. HPCs in turn generate a range of more differentiated cells and ultimately all the blood cell lineages (Figure 1). The process of haematopoiesis is exquisitely regulated in health with a homeostatic balance maintained between numbers produced and those undergoing programmed cell death (apoptosis).

HSCs are pluripotent while HPCs are multipotent and eventually following a number of cell division episodes become committed to given lineages i.e. red blood cells, leukocytes and platelets. The system is highly prolific with one HSC being capable of producing approximately 10^6 mature blood cells following 20 sequential divisions.

In the early foetus the yolk sac is the main site of haematopoiesis, from around 6 weeks until 6-7 months of gestation, haematopoiesis occurs in the liver and spleen. The bone marrow takes over as the major site of haematopoiesis thereafter with the entire bone marrow being haematopoietic during childhood. Haematopoietic tissue recedes towards adulthood and is ultimately confined to the proximal ends of the long bones, vertebral column, sternum and pelvic girdle in the adult.

Within the active bone marrow space, a supportive microenvironment exists which is composed of stromal cells of various types. These stromal cells secrete and also sequester molecules such as growth factors that support haematopoiesis.

13.2 More about Haematopoietic Stem Cells and Progenitor Cells

A major thrust of basic HSC research since the 1960s has the identification and characterisation these stem cells. This has been difficult because HSCs look morphologically like other immature white blood cells. However, certain key protein markers discriminate between HSCs and other cell types. Only about 1 in every 10,000 bone marrow cells is thought to be a genuine stem cell. In the blood stream the proportion falls to 1 in 100,000 blood cells. Early in vitro experimental work used mouse models where murine bone marrow cells were injected into recipient mice that had received irradiation sufficient to kill their own blood-producing cells. If the recipients recovered and all types of blood cells reappeared (bearing a genetic marker from the donor animal), the transplanted cells would be deemed to have included haematopoietic stem cells. These studies revealed that there appear to be two kinds of HSCs. If bone marrow cells from the transplanted mouse can, in turn, be transplanted to another lethally irradiated mouse to restore its haematopoietic system these cells are considered *long-term progenitor cells* capable of self renewal., Multipotent and committed HPCs capable of regenerating all the different types of blood cells, cannot renew themselves over the long term so these are referred to as *short-term progenitor cells.*

More contemporary research has shown that it is possible to demonstrate long term self renewal, proliferation and differentiation in *vitro* using haematopoietic cell culture techniques. Haematopoietic progenitor cells inoculated into cell culture flasks pre-prepared with irradiated stromal cell feeder layers can give rise to pluripotent HSCs, multipotent HPCs and differentiated haematopoietic cells of all the blood type lineages (Figure 2)

Progenitor cells are relatively immature cells that are precursors to a fully differentiated cell of the same tissue type. They are capable of proliferating, but they have a limited capacity to differentiate into more than one cell type as HSCs do. A stem cell however, is capable of self-renewal as it must be able to renew itself for the entire lifespan of the organism. It is these long-term replicating HSCs that are most important for developing HSC-based cell therapies. See Chapter 11 for more information about stem cell biology.

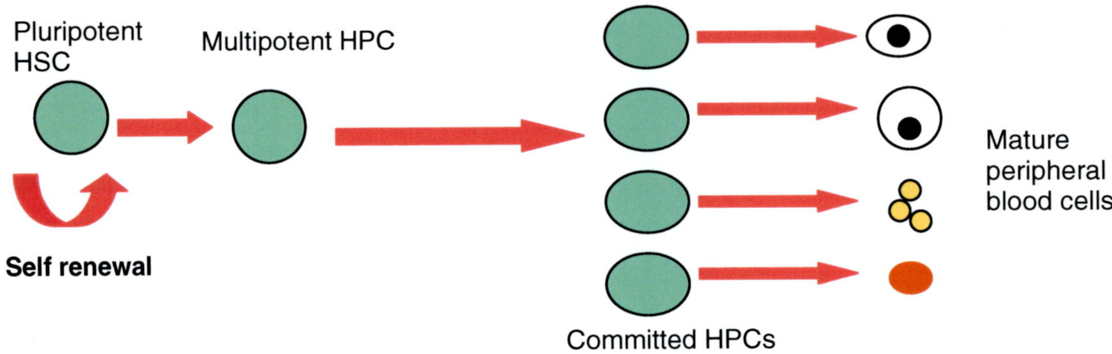

Figure 1: Schematic diagram of haematopoiesis showing progression from HSC through HPC stages of development to mature peripheral blood cell formation.

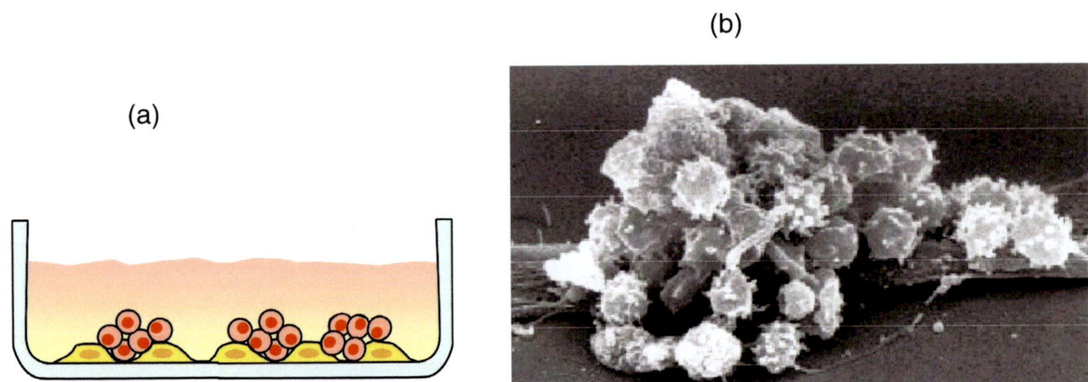

Figure 2 (a) Diagramatic representation of a longterm invitro culture of HSCs and HPCs *in vitro* (b) Scanning electron micrograph of a colony of haematopoietic cells in culture

13.3 Haematopoietic Cells for Therapeutic Use

Historically "haematopoietic stem cell transplantation" has been the term used to describe the therapeutic use of these cells. Although the term is still commonly used, more recently the terminology has been modified and unified by the Joint Accreditation Committee-International Society for Cellular Therapy & European Group for Blood and Marrow Transplantation (JACIE) Haematopoietic Progenitor Cell (HPC) is now the preferred term but in much of the literature "stem" cells are still referred to.

There is further discussion about the characteristics of stem cells in Chapter 11.

13.3.1 Bone Marrow

Historically HPCs have been bone marrow aspirated directly from the bone marrow space within the posterior iliac crests and sternum of donors while under general anaesthetic. As mentioned above, about 1 in every 10,000 cells in the marrow is a pluripotent HSC or HPC, but other cells harvested include multipotent and committed HPCs, stromal cells and mature and maturing white and red blood cells. Typically 500-1500mls of bone marrow is collected. A mononuclear count is taken to determine the yield which should be around $2\text{-}4\text{x}10^8$ /kg body weight of the recipient. Harvested bone marrow must be processed aseptically to yield the buffy coat or mononuclear cell fraction – the process is described in Chapter 6. The accepted abbreviation for marrow derived HPCs is HPC, Marrow.

13.3.2 Peripheral Blood

The use of bone marrow as a source of HPCs (HPC, Marrow) has become much less prevalent over the last 10 years with peripheral blood HPCs now being the preferred source. It is possible to coax or mobilise HPCs from the bone marrow space by a variety of regimens. In the case of a normal donor, the growth factor granulocyte colony stimulating factor (G-CSF) is generally used to boost HPC production and to cause adhesion molecule bonds holding the cells in the bone marrow space to be released. If mobilisation is successful, HPCs are released into the peripheral blood from where they can be harvested using apheresis techniques, thus the abbreviation for these cells is HPC, Apheresis.

In the case autologous transplantation where the patient donates cells for their own use, the mobilisation process generally involves administration of chemotherapy followed by G-CSF. If on the other hand, an allogeneic donor is being used, the mobilisation protocol uses only G-CSF. There is currently considerable research underway to look at improving mobilisation.

Plerixafor is a novel stem cell mobilising agent that reversibly inhibits the interaction of CXCR-4 and SDF1-alpha, releasing stem cells from the marrow. Plerixafor is a subcutaneous agent that is administered at 10.00pm the night before beginning commencement of stem cell collection. Thus administration needs to be coordinated with the apheresis procedure.

Following successful mobilisation, the apheresis process involves use of either an intravenous cannula or catheter to remove blood from the donor (approximately 300mls at a time) and centrifugation of the blood to yield different fractions based on specific gravity. The mononuclear cell fraction which contains the HPCs is extracted and the other cellular and plasma components returned to the donor. Typically 2 to 3 total blood volumes will be processed per apheresis procedure. The process of apheresis is described in Chapter 14.

13.3.3 Umbilical Cord Blood

In the late 1980s and early 1990s, scientists began to recognise that blood from the human umbilical cord and placenta was a rich source of HPCs. The umbilical cord is usually discarded at birth. Since the first successful umbilical cord blood transplants in children with Fanconi anaemia, the collection and therapeutic use of these cells has grown quickly.

Umbilical cord blood banks such as those in New York and NHSBT in Bristol (the NHS-Cord Blood Bank) have over 500,000 cord blood donations available worldwide for transplantation into patients who need HPCs. The volumes of cord blood collections mean the recipients are usually children although more recently 2 or even 3 cord blood units have been used together to transplant adults. Internationally thousands of cord blood units have been supplied to patients. There is a substantial amount of research being conducted on cord blood to explore the possibility of ex vivo expansion and to further characterise the unique properties and therapeutic potential of this valuable resource. The accepted abbreviation for cord blood derived HPCs is HPC, Cord Blood. There is more detail about cord blood banking in Chapter 16.

Table 1. Relative advantages and disadvantages of different HPC sources

Source	Advantages	Disadvantages
Bone marrow	No stem cell mobilisation required	Requires general anaesthetic Few days off work May render donor temporarily anaemic Pain following harvest at aspiration sites.
Peripheral blood	Ease of collection No general anaesthetic Attain high stem cell doses Faster engraftment after HPCT Return to work on day post harvesting	Requires stem cell mobilisation with growth factor +/- chemotherapy May require central venous catheter if inadequate peripheral access Hypocalcaemia during apheresis
Cord blood	Widely available Ease of collection less GvHD than with HPC, Marrow or HPC, Apheresis	Low volumes therefore lower HPC dose Not being able to return to donor for donor lymphocytes High cost of establishing a cord blood bank

Key:
HPC: Haematopoietic progenitor cells
HPCT: Haematopoietic progenitor cell transplantation
GvHD: Graft vs. Host Disease

13.3.4 Assessing the Haematopoietic Progenitor Cell Content of Stem Cell Collections

It is important to be able to enumerate HPCs in HPC, Apheresis, HPC, Marrow or HPC, Cord Blood collections in order to determine the dose available to the patient. The marker typically used to identify HPCs is CD34, which is a cell surface antigen expressed on these cells. Flow cytometric assessment of CD34 positivity is carried out on samples from harvested cells to determine the yield of HPCs. In the case of HPC, Apheresis cells more than one harvesting episode may be required to achieve an adequate HPC dose of at least 2×10^6 CD34 positive cells per kg for the recipient. With HPC, Cord Blood and HPC, Marrow products, only one collection is possible so the cell dose obtained cannot be readily augmented.

In patients or donors undergoing mobilisation regimens as discussed above it is common practice to commence daily assessment of CD34 positivity in the peripheral blood after approximately 5 days of administration of G-CSF. The decision to commence harvesting is usually based on a peripheral blood count of 10 CD34 positive cells/µl.

There is more information on HPC collections in Chapter 14 while flow cytometry is described in Chapter 15.

13.4 Autologous Haematopoietic Progenitor Cell Transplantation

Autologous transplantation involves the collection of HPCs from the patient themselves and subsequent re-infusion following high dose chemotherapy +/- radiotherapy. Chemotherapy and radiotherapy are associated with several adverse effects including immunosuppression and damage to haematopoietic function within the bone marrow a result of which, treatment-associated morbidity and mortality can be significant. The possible occurrence of secondary cancers, possibly years after the transplant treatment, is of great concern. These side effects are particularly apparent following the high dose regimens that are often given to patients – the aim of which is to destroy as much tumour as possible.

The rationale behind autologous HPCT is to use the patient's own HPC, Marrow or HPC, Apheresis cells to reconstitute haematopoiesis and thus "rescue" the patient after the administration of escalated doses of chemo- and/or radiotherapy. Transplant-related mortality (TRM) is much lower in autologous (1-5% in most series) than allogeneic HPCT so these procedures can be performed in patients up to 65-70 years of age.

One potential major drawback associated with autologous transplantation is the possibility of disease relapse due to contaminating tumour cells in the graft Even following several courses of chemotherapy, the patient may still have minimal residual disease present which is almost or completely undetectable even by molecular means. If such malignant cells are harvested and re-infused they may outrun the recovery of normal haematopoietic tissue meaning that the patient will relapse.

It is worth bearing in mind that although often successful, autologous HPC transplantation is not always curative and this is accepted in certain cases where the procedure can halt the disease progression for a time but does not represent a cure.

Autologous HPCs are mostly collected for transplantation as part of a planned treatment protocol. Typically, cells are processed and stored in an accredited laboratory. The harvested cells undergo careful cryopreservation and storage in vapour phase nitrogen using practices and procedures designed to optimise cell integrity and viability. Patients usually undergo the transplant process within a few weeks/months of HPC harvesting and storage but occasionally their cells can be banked for future use. Such collections are sometimes termed "rainy day" harvests and are used if the patient's disease relapses at a later stage or as "back up" for a planned allogeneic transplant in case of graft rejection. See Chapter 15 for a description of cell cryopreservation and storage.

13.5 Allogeneic Haematopoietic Progenitor Cell Transplantation

Non-self or allogeneic donors are either siblings, relatives or may be unrelated volunteer donors (VUDs). Donor selection is based on HLA typing and fitness to donate (Chapter 17). Typically, partially HLA-matched related haploidentical (parent/sibling) or HLA-matched unrelated volunteer donors (VUDs) are used as a source of HSCs. If more than one HLA-identical donor is available factors considered in donor selection are CMV serology, age, blood group and gender.

Most VUDs are found via searching national and international donor registries such as the British Bone Marrow Registry (BBMR), the Anthony Nolan or other donor programmes. It is usual to aim for an allogeneic HPC, Apheresis or HPC, Marrow harvest collection of around 4×10^6 CD34 positive HPCs per kg of the recipient's weight. Cord blood banks enhance the available donor pool, especially for ethnic minorities whose HLA phenotypes are under-represented in the current bone marrow registries Cord blood units are selected on both tissue type match, total nucleated cell (TNC) dose and CD34 count where available. The minimum recommendations for patients with malignant diseases are for 3×10^7 and 2×10^7 TNC and CD34 /kg patient body weight respectively with a 4 out of 6 HLA match. Increasing the cord blood cell dose abrogates the influence of the HLA mismatches. In non-malignant diseases the recommendation is for a higher cell dose of 4.9×10^7 TNC/kg. In situations, particularly in the adult setting, where a single CB unit is insufficient to meet the recommended cell dose, double CB transplants (2 units administered sequentially) are being used. Both CB units are selected to match both the recipient and each other, and the cumulative cell dose must be adequate.

13.5.1 Graft vs. Host Disease and Graft vs. Malignancy Effect

Whatever the source, allogeneic HPCs can not only reconstitute the haematopoietic and immune systems after high dose chemotherapy which is given to destroy the tumour in the recipient but are also capable of mounting a potent graft vs. malignancy (GvM) effect. In essence this is immunotherapy *in vivo* and is a major benefit of allogeneic transplantation. Historically, the GvM phenomenon was referred to as Graft vs. Leukaemia (GvL) effect as it was first noted in leukaemic patients. Both terms GvM and GvL are used today although strictly speaking the former is more appropriate.

This very valuable GvM effect is mediated primarily by immunocompetent T lymphocytes in the graft recognising and attacking malignant cells in the recipient. There is also the very real possibility of donor lymphocytes attacking non-malignant host tissues and organs as they are perceived as "non-self". This complication is termed Graft vs. Host Disease (GvHD). GvHD is mediated by donor cytotoxic CD8+ lymphocytes and lymphokine-secreting CD4+ T helper lymphocytes in the graft.

These cells are activated by major and minor histoincompatibilities between donor and recipient and are fuelled by the cytokine storm (released as a result of chemotherapy) generating a cascade of inflammatory mediators. The severity of GvHD is linked to the degree of HLA mismatch between the donor and recipient therefore HLA typing and matching is a critical issue in donor selection. See Chapter 17 for a detailed description of HLA typing and transplantation. The ideal scenario would involve the use of a closely matched donor and recipient but with minor histocompatibility antigen disparities to minimise the chances of GvHD but at the same time allow for a GvM effect. It is possible to manipulate harvested donor HPCs ex vivo to selectively remove subpopulations of cells responsible for GvHD using monoclonal antibody based techniques. These technologies are described in detail in Chapter 15.

GvHD typically affects the skin, gut and liver and can be divided into two distinct clinical entities: acute GvHD typically occurring within the first 100 days of the HSCT and manifesting as a rash, erythroderma, diarrhoea, paralytic ileus and jaundice and chronic GvHD which onsets after day 100 and resembles an autoimmune disease with sclerodermatous skin changes, malabsorption and obstructive jaundice. The most dangerous effect of both types of GvHD is the profound immunosuppression resulting from the GvHD process itself and from agents used to treat GvHD.

Prevention of GvHD is generally more successful than treatment once the condition is established. T-cell depletion of the graft successfully reduces the incidence and severity of GvHD but is associated with a concomitant increase in the incidence of graft rejection, disease relapse and delayed immunological reconstitution. The alternative approach is the use of immunosuppressive agents such as cyclosporin A and methotrexate post-transplant. Corticosteroids are the first-line agents in the treatment of GvHD and anti-thymocyte globulin can be used as salvage therapy in acute GvHD. Chronic GvHD may be difficult to treat, Cyclosporin A having limited efficacy in this setting. Alternative approaches include mycophenolate, thalidomide and extracorporeal photopheresis. Most of these agents compound the risk of infection in these patients but on the other hand, moderate-severe GvHD confers a high risk of morbidity and mortality.

Table 2. Evidence for an Allogeneic Graft vs. Malignancy Effect

Evidence
Reduced risk of leukaemia relapse in patients with acute and chronic GvHD
Increased risk of relapse after syngeneic (identical twin) transplants
Increased risk of relapse after T-cell depleted transplants
Demonstration of donor-derived T-cell clones reactive against neoplastic cells
Reintroduction of remission by DLI in patients relapsing post-allogeneic HPCT

Key
GvHD: graft versus host disease
DLI: donor lymphocyte infusion
HPCT: haematopoietic progenitor cell transplant

13.5.2 Chimerism Following Allogeneic Transplantation

The balance of donor and recipient haematopoietic and immune cells in the months post transplant are closely monitored in blood and bone marrow samples taken from the recipient at intervals. Ideally the recipient haematopoietic and immune systems become totally replaced by donor cells. In the interim, while this change is happening, the host is described as "chimeric". The chimeric status of the host is assessed by DNA and or polymorphism studies to identify exactly what percentage of their HPCs are donor or recipient derived. The aim is to achieve 100% donor status. Falling or unstable chimerism where the haematopoietic/immune systems revert back to recipient are generally a sign of failing graft or relapse.

13.6 Pre-Transplant Preparative Regimens

Before infusion of autologous or allogeneic HPCs the patient is likely to be treated with high doses of chemotherapy and/or radiotherapy as mentioned above. There are three aims of this so-called conditioning regimen:

1. The destruction of any residual malignant cells

2. The creation of 'space' for the new stem cells to grow

3. Immunosuppression to prevent destruction of the allograft by any residual immunologically competent recipient cells

The choice of conditioning regimen depends on the patient's disease and the degree of histocompatibility of the stem cells. Typically, conditioning regimens are very cytotoxic and are associated with significant side effects. Transplant related mortality (TRM) is a very real concern. Side effects are summarised in Table 3.

Table 3 Side effects associated with high dose chemotherapy/radiotherapy

Side effects associated with pre-transplant conditioning
Hair loss
Myelosuppression
Immunosuppression
Gastro-intestinal problems i.e. mucositis
Infertility
Secondary cancers

13.6.1 Reduced Intensity Conditioning

As mentioned above, it is well recognised that a significant part of the "curative" effect of allogeneic HPC transplantation is immune-mediated - the so-called Graft vs. Malignancy (GvM) or Graft vs. Leukaemia (GvL) effect. Clinicians have recently developed a strategy of exploiting the GvM phenomenon. This therapeutic option involves the short term administration of well tolerated immunosuppressive agents rather than using high dose chemotherapy/radiotherapy. These non-myeloablative regimens, termed "mini" or "reduced intensity conditioning (RIC)" transplants include agents such as fludarabine, antithymocyte globulin (ATG) and busulphan and its analogues and sometimes lower dose radiotherapy. The aim is to reduce transplant related morbidity and mortality whilst providing sufficient immunosuppression to allow engraftment of transplanted allogeneic HPCs which include a large number of immunocompetent T lymphocytes capable of mediating GvM. The reduced TRM increases the applicability of RIC HPCTs to older patients or patients with co-morbid disease.

Patients may receive infusions of additional donor lymphocyte (DLI) at a later stage to augment the GvM effect but with caution because GvHD is a significant complication of such transplants. The accepted term used to describe a therapeutic cell product containing a quantified T cell population is T Cells Therapeutic (TC-T). TC-T infusion doses are carefully worked out on the basis of the CD3 content of the harvested cells. Appropriate doses are administered to patients based on the degree of relapse or chimeric status.

13.7 Clinical Indications for the Use of Haematopoietic Progenitor Cells

There is an ever increasing range of conditions that can be treated with autologous or allogeneic transplantation using HPCs sourced from bone marrow, mobilised peripheral blood or cord blood. Some of the main indications are described below.

13.7.1 Haematological Malignancies

The main clinical use of HSCs has always been in the treatment of haematological malignancies which are cancers of the blood, bone marrow and lymphoid tissues (table 4). These include the leukaemias, lymphomas and multiple myeloma among others. These malignancies are clonal in origin and arise from flaws in the genetic make-up of progenitor cells in the bone marrow or lymphoid tissue resulting in uncontrolled proliferation, failure to mature properly and failure to undergo programmed cell death appropriately. The malignant cells can overwhelm the bone marrow space and lymphoid tissues and spill into the peripheral blood. Autologous or allogeneic transplantation are treatment options which are used to treat these diseases following careful consideration by clinicians The transplant process has been described in detail above but briefly, the cancerous haematopoietic cells are destroyed via radiation or chemotherapy, followed by infusion of the patient's own (autologous) or donor (allogeneic) HPCs. An added benefit provided by allogeneic transplantation is the GvM effect.

13.7.2 Solid Tumours

Therapy for non-haematological solid tumours may include autologous HPC transplantation. The rationale is the same as for the treatment of the haematological malignancies – high dose chemotherapy/radiotherapy is administered to destroy the tumour but an inevitable side effect of this treatment is destruction of the haematopoietic and immune systems. Previously harvested and stored autologous HPCs are used to rescue the patients' bone marrow function. Tumours treated in the manner include germ cell tumours, Ewing's sarcoma, neuroblastoma, meduloblastoma.

13.7.3 Other Indications

Another use of allogeneic HPC transplants is in the treatment of hereditary blood disorders. Different types of inherited anaemia (failure to produce red blood cells) fall into this category of diseases and include: aplastic anaemia, beta-thalassemia, Blackfan-Diamond syndrome, sickle-cell anaemia, severe combined immunodeficiency and Wiskott-Aldrich syndrome.

Also treatable by allogeneic transplantation are inborn errors of metabolism (genetic disorders characterised by defects in key enzymes need to produce essential body components or degrade chemical by-products). These disorders include: Hurler's syndrome, Lesch Nyhan syndrome, Hunter's syndrome and Gaucher's disease. There has been some success in treating certain autoimmune conditions such as Lupus Erythematosis and Multiple Sclerosis with autologous transplantation. Because HPC transplantation has a high risk of attendant transplant related morbidity and mortality this treatment option is not undertaken lightly and is often used as a last resort.

Table 4. Indications for Haematopoietic Progenitor Cell Transplantation

Disease	Preferred Type of HSCT
Acute myeloid leukaemias	Allogeneic; autologous if no fully matched sibling/donor
Acute lymphoblastic leukaemias	Allogeneic
Chronic myeloid leukaemia	Allogeneic
Chronic lymphocytic leukaemia	Allogeneic in patients over 40yrs
Non-Hodgkin's lymphoma histologically aggressive	Autologous in most cases except in B cell Acute lymphoblastic leukaemia and anaplastic CD20 negative disease.
Non-Hodgkin's lymphoma -histologically indolent	Autologous in most cases
Hodgkin's disease	Autologous in most cases
Multiple Myeloma	Autologous in most cases but allogeneic transplants now being considered
Severe aplastic anaemia	Allogeneic
Breast cancer	Autologous but controversial
Haemoglobinopathies	Allogeneic
Immune deficiency syndromes	Allogeneic
Autoimmune Diseases	Autologous
Metabolic disorders	Allogeneic

(Please note that this is not an exhaustive list)

13.7.4 Benefits and Complications of autologous and allogeneic Haematopoietic Progenitor Cell Transplantation

Autologous and allogeneic transplant procedures are potentially curative therapeutic options in some cases but nonetheless the relative benefits and drawbacks must be weighed up for each individual by clinicians, the patients themselves and their relatives. The tables below summarise the main comparative aspects of these treatment options.

Table 5a   Benefits Associated with Autologous HPC Transplantation

Factor	Benefit
No donor search needed	Less delay in commencing treatment
Self-self	No rejection, no GvHD
Associated with less morbidity and mortality than allografting	Less time in hospital with fewer complications and faster haematopoietic recovery; appropriate for older patients and those with co-morbidities

Table 5b Complications Associated with Autologous HPC Transplantation

Cause	Early Complications	Late Complications
Regimen-related	Mucositis; cardiac and renal, impairment, haemorrhagic cystitis; neurological problems.	Endocrine related growth failure; thyroid disease; osteoporosis; infertility; cataracts. Long term damage to HPCs
Haematopoietic/ Immune	Delayed or failed engraftment	Delayed haematopoietic and immune reconstitution.
Self-Self	Infusion of cancer cells	Relapse
Infections	Viral; bacterial; fungal.	Bacterial, fungal, viral.
Other	Failure to mobilise HPCs	Transplant not an option

Table 6a   Benefits Associated with Allogeneic HPC Transplantation

Factor	Benefit
Donor cells used	GvM effect; able to treat certain non-malignant conditions
Possibility of RIC allograft	Less time in hospital with fewer complications; appropriate for older patients and those with co-morbidities
High intensity conditioning	Chance of "cure" in patients able to tolerate therapy

Table 6b Complications Associated with Allogeneic HPC Transplantation

Cause	Early Complications	Late Complications
Regimen-related	.Mucositis; cardiac and renal, impairment, haemorrhagic cystitis; neurological problems.	Endocrine related growth failure; thyroid disease; osteoporosis; infertility; cataracts. Long term damage to HPCs
Haematopoietic / Immune	Graft rejection; graft failure; acute GvHD.	Graft failure; chronic GvHD; delayed haematopoietic and immune reconstitution.
Infections	Viral; bacterial; fungal.	Bacterial, fungal, viral.
Pulmonary	Interstitial pneumonitis; diffuse alveolar haemorrhage.	Bronchioloitis obliterans.
Other	Hepatic venocclusive disease; thrombotic microangiopathy, gastrointestinal problems	Secondary malignancies.

13.8 Summary and Future Perspectives

There is an important role for the use of autologous and allogeneic transplantation in malignant and non-malignant conditions in adults and paediatric patients. Advances in our understanding the biology of HPCs combined with technical improvements have been significant over the past few years. The indications for HPCT are likely to increase therefore we must continue to work to optimise and refine these therapeutic options.

HPC mobilisation is an area where a great deal of attention is currently focussed. The advent of novel agents such as Plerixafor that can cleave the bonds between the bone marrow stromal micro-environment and HPCs even in previous poor mobilisers is of great interest. We are gaining more expertise in the therapeutic use of cord blood HPCs with encouraging results. The proposed expansion of cord blood banking is a tantalising development as the full potential of HPC-Cs is not yet fully understood. The use of RIC regimens has extended the use of allogeneic transplantation to older patients and those with co-morbidities that would otherwise have precluded an allogeneic procedure. These more innovative approaches to HPCT are currently well underway but it is perhaps in the field of "stem cell plasticity" that we will see the most exciting advances (See Chapter 81). Research is indicating that HPCs may not be as restricted in their developmental potential as we previously thought and this is leading to the possibility of using these cells in regenerative medicine.

13.9 Suggested Reading

1. A comprehensive overview of stem cell biology can be found at
    http://stemcells.nih.gov/.

2. NETCORD-FACT International Standards Accreditation Manual Third Edition

3. S. Querol et al Haematologica (2009); doi: 10.3324/haematol. (2008).002741
    Cord blood stem cells for hematopoietic stem cell transplantation in the UK:
    how big should the bank be?

4. Panagiotis et al. Haematologica Journal, (2006), 91:852-855
    A non-myeloablative conditioning regimen in allogeneic stem cell
    transplantation from related and unrelated donors in elderly patients

5. J. F. DiPersio et al. Blood; Pre published online Apr 10, 2009;
    doi:10.1182/blood-2008-08-174946 Plerixafor and G-CSF versus placebo and
    G-CSF to mobilize hematopoietic stem cells for autologous stem cell
    transplantation in patients with multiple myeloma

6. WEB SOURCE:

    http://www.marrow.org/PHYSICIAN/Adv_in_Auto_Allo_Tx/Hematopoietic_Cell_
    Sources_Tai/index.html

7. V Rocha et al New England Journal of Medicine (2004) 351; 2276-2285

8. Transplants of Umbilical-Cord Blood or Bone Marrow from Unrelated Donors
    in Adults with Acute Leukemia

9. JACIE WEB SITE http://www.jacie.org/

10. Romeo A. Graft Versus Host Disease Medscape article:

    http://emedicine.medscape.com/article/429037-overview

11. Thomas' Hematopoietic Cell Transplantation. 3rd edn. Blume KG, Forman SJ,
    Appelbaum FR. (eds). Pages 16 to 30.

12. The Clinical Practice of Stem Cell Transplantation. Barrett J, Treleaven J.
    (eds). Isis Medical Media (1998).

13. Haemopoietic Stem Cell Transplantation. The EBMT Handbook (2004).
    Apperley J, Carreras E, Gluckman E, Gratwohl A, Masszi T (eds). Pages 79 –
    106; 133 – 146, 163 – 196.

14. Practical Hemopoietic Stem Cell Transplantation. Cant A J, Galoway A,
    Jackson G (eds). Pages 23 – 40; 117 – 125.

15. Cellular Therapy. A Physician's Handbook. Snyder EL, Haley NR (eds). Pages
    103 – 135.

13.10 Self Assessment Questions

Multiple Choice Questions

1. Which of the following statements about HPCT are true?
   a) HPCs must always be mobilised from the bone marrow space for harvesting
   b) The therapeutic use of HPC-A products is more prevalent than HPC-M or HPC-C
   c) HPCT is appropriate for some non-malignant conditions
   d) HPC-A transplants are associated with more GvHD than HPC-C transplants
   e) HPCs are can be identified using flow cytometric assessment of CD34 expression

2. Allogeneic stem cell donors are selected on the basis of:
   a) HLA match for recipient
   b) CMV status
   c) Physical fitness
   d) Blood group
   e) Ethnic background

3. Which of the following statements about GvHD are true?
   a) GvHD is mediated by CD4 and CD8 T cells
   b) GVHD is always a chronic disorder
   c) Matching donor and recipient at major HLA loci will prevent GvHD
   d) GvHD and GvM are mediated by similar mechanisms
   e) Tends to be less severe following transplantation of cord blood stem cells

4. Which of the following statements are true of reduced intensity conditioning allogeneic transplants?
   a) They are associated with lower transplant-related mortality than regimens using high dose conditioning
   b) They may be considered in patients with co-morbid diseases
   c) They owe their efficacy to the use of myeloablative drugs
   d) They are associated with a higher incidence of relapse
   e) They may allow stem cell transplantation in older patients

Short Answer Questions

1. Describe the advantages and disadvantages of cord blood as a source of haematopoietic stem cells

2. Describe the process of normal haematopoiesis.

Assignments

1. Compare and contrast autologous and allogeneic transplantation for haematological malignancies – explaining the relative benefits and drawbacks of each therapeutic option.

2. If you were a clinician how would you explain the steps involved in mobilisation, harvesting, storage and ultimate use of peripheral blood progenitor cells to a patient about to undergo the process for autologous transplantation?

14 COLLECTION OF HAEMATOPOIETIC PROGENITOR CELLS (HPC)

14.1 Referrals

Written referral is required for all stem cell collections to be processed. It is important that the clinical team signs a written prescription specifying the exact procedures to be performed for any given product. Collection dates should be agreed with the processing laboratory to avoid excessive workload. It must be signed by a responsible member of the clinical team and must be in accordance with service level agreements. Collections may be made by a third party. The responsibilities of that third party, and those of the stem cell laboratory must be understood. A robust chain of communication is needed from clinician through collection to processing.

Donors and patients awaiting HPC, Apheresis or HPC, Marrow harvesting must be tested for current mandatory markers, including HIV, Hepatitis B & C, HTLV and Syphilis, at less than 30 days prior to the proposed harvest date. Donor testing is considered further in Chapter 5. This will identify infectious donors and enable the clinical team and the laboratory to plan ahead for handling any product found positive. These tests will be repeated on all products at collection. It is important that the sample is not bled more than 30 days prior to the harvest date to minimise 'window' period infection. Close liaison is required with the clinical and collection teams to anticipate complex referrals and resolve any incidents consequent on collection.

14.2 Bone Marrow Harvesting

14.2.1 Timing and Co-ordination

Bone marrow harvesting in an operating theatre requires organisation. Booking of theatre, preparation of the patient, consent, collection and availability of cross matched blood, booking anaesthetist and collection staff and preparation of kit, all need to be organised. Target yields links between patient and donor and other specific requirements need to be prescribed by the referring clinician. The patient or donor will have been counselled, examined and tested to ensure fitness for the anaesthetic and suitability for the transplant.

14.2.2 Role of Healthcare Scientist

This may vary from no role at all, where marrow is collected by a third party to a major role in organisation and preparation of the collection kit. Technical staff need to be familiar with SOPs, both for their own unit and for third parties. Where third parties are involved, service level agreements must specify the roles of all parties and parameters relating to products.

14.2.3 Operating Theatre Environment

The donor or patient will be anaesthetised with their posterior ileac crests exposed for multiple punctures using large bore needles. Two operators on either side of the patient aspirate small volumes of marrow at each puncture into heparinised syringes. These are then pooled into an anti-coagulated collection bag. Healthcare Scientists attending operating theatres must be familiar with local Trust operating theatre protocols for scrubbing, gowning up and other aseptic techniques. Preparation of equipment may be performed partly prior to entering the operating theatre, depending on local procedure. Collected marrow will be filtered through a series of filters to remove large particles of bone clots and other tissue. These filters may block and require replacement.

14.2.4 Preparation of Anticoagulant

Preservative-free heparin or other specified anticoagulant is required for washing and priming syringes and for priming the collection bag to prevent clotting. It is important that adequate volumes and concentrations are prepared to local procedures. Adequate anticoagulation throughout the collection is necessary to maximise yield.

Collection sets vary but include anti-coagulated syringes, disposable bone marrow aspiration needles, collection bags, coarse and finer filters and sample tubes. These need to be prepared to SOP. A Healthcare Scientist may be involved in the preparation of equipment, injection of filled syringes into the collection bag, changing blocked filters, washing and priming syringes and assisting collection staff. This will all be covered by local SOPs.

14.2.5 Cell Counts and Volumes

Local procedures will specify an approximate target volume. Patients will have a specified target nucleated cell yield. Generally, after about half of the projected volume has been collected (around 600mls), a sample will be taken from the collection bag and sent to the haematology laboratory. The target collection volume necessary to achieve the target nucleated cell yield will then be calculated according to charts relating bone marrow nucleated cell concentration to recipient's weight. The collection will then proceed until an adequate volume is in the bag. Collection filters may need to be changed if blocked. Final samples should be specified before the harvest. A maximum safe collection volume will be specified.

Children will donate smaller volumes. It is important that maximum permitted volumes as specified by local procedures are not exceeded. Calculation of target volume to achieve target cell yield requires careful calculation, particularly where there are large differentials in recipient and donor weight.

14.2.6 Labelling and Transport

After filtration of the product, this will need to be labelled using unique identifiers, to local protocol. Any samples and accompanying documentation will need to be labelled. Validated transport containers will need to be used to enable transportation at 4°C to the processing laboratory.

14.3 Peripheral Blood Stem Cell Harvesting by Apheresis

14.3.1 Timing

HPC, Apheresis harvesting requires mobilisation of stem cells from marrow to peripheral blood. G-CSF with or without chemotherapy will be given 5 to7 days prior to the estimated date of harvest. The patient's underlying condition, conditioning chemotherapy, the timing and dose of G-CSF all affect the prediction of the harvest date but this is often imprecise. Healthcare Scientists need to be prepared for variable workload and adjust the cases taken on accordingly. Peripheral blood taken from the donor or patient prior to harvest and assayed for total white count, MNC and CD34+ concentrations will inform on the best harvest date. There is a close correlation between the peripheral blood CD34+ concentration (cells/microlitre) and the yield of CD34+ cells in the harvest. HPC, Apheresis harvest would not generally commence (be initiated) until the CD34+ concentration exceeds 10 cells/microlitre. It is important that Healthcare Scientists are familiar with and closely involved in communication and are informed of decisions to harvest. Protocols need to be clear and communication efficient regarding the need for harvests on subsequent days. Staff will be informed when the target yield has been achieved, or if a decision has been made that cells have not mobilised adequately.

The target yield will have been specified prior to harvesting. It will generally be in the order of 2 to 5 x 10e6/Kg for autologous recipients and will generally exceed 4x10e9/Kg recipient weight.

14.3.2 Principles of Collection by Apheresis

The patient/donor will have been prepared, counselled and consented as above. Vascular access will enable flow into and back from the apheresis machine. The machine will separate buffy coat from red cell and plasma fractions and collect a white cell concentrate containing bone marrow progenitors. Different apheresis technologies and different programmes will affect the volume, concentration, speed and reliability of peripheral blood stem cell collections. These include manual programmes, requiring subjective intervention by apheresis staff, or automated programmes generally requiring less operator intervention. Apheresis staff experience, procedure times and the volume of blood processed by the apheresis machine will all affect the yield. Procedural problems such as poor mobilisation of stem cells, failure to find the red cell/plasma interface, poor venous flow and incomplete collection will similarly affect yield. Extending the procedure time to process more blood may enable an adequate collection but will delay the start of processing. It is important that Healthcare Scientists are familiar with the circumstances and problems faced by collection teams and are in close communication with them. Clinical information from the collection team must be recorded, particularly if related to Central Venous Catheter or other sepsis which may affect product validation.

14.3.3 Sampling

Mandatory microbiology and bacteriology samples, cell counts, CFUGM and other samples need to be specified prior to the harvest and adequately labelled to protocol. Poor handling of samples may delay processing.

14.3.4 Labelling and Documentation

Collection bags, samples and documentation all need to be labelled using unique identifiers to protocol. Spare labels will need to be accounted for. Healthcare Scientists need to be familiar with procedures for transportation and service level agreements where collection is performed by a third party.

14.3.5 Products

Generally, an apheresis machine will concentrate circulating nucleated cells and increase the percentage of CD34+ cells. This is generally achieved after processing between 2 and 3 blood volumes over 3½ hours. Autologous plasma is generally collected to a similar volume to the white cell concentrate to enable the dilution of cryoprotectant. This is usually done towards the end of the procedure. Clinical problems may make plasma collection difficult, requiring the use of an alternative diluent such as Human Albumin Solution.

14.3.6 Patients and Donors

This is a reliable collection method in children (to 10kgs and below) resulting in similar yields when adjusted to recipient weight. Paediatric collections may need to involve priming of the apheresis machine using irradiated compatible donor red cells.

14.3.7 Donor Lymphocyte Harvest

Donor derived T Lymphocytes may be required for infusion after the transplant to treat relapse. These cells are labelled TC-T Cells. They may be collected as part of the original harvest or as a separate apheresis procedure, performed some weeks or months after allogeneic transplantation. The donor is not stimulated by G-CSF and the dose of CD3 positive T lymphocytes collected is hard to predict.

Generally, the collection will be aliquoted to the clinician's prescription into sequentially increasing CD3 doses. The smallest dose will probably be returned, uncryopreserved, on the day of collection for immediate infusion. Donors will have been prepared for this at counselling. All mandatory testing needs to be repeated.

14.3.8 Therapeutic Leucopheresis

Newly diagnosed leukaemia patients may require leucoreduction to treat leucostasis (very high white cell concentration threatening infarction, ischaemia or death). Historically, in this situation it may have been seen as advantageous to store cells. Many of these cells are capable of bone marrow reconstitution should the patient's disease progress at a later stage. This is no longer recommended in current guidance but the stem cell laboratory may have been asked to cryopreserve a fraction of the very large number of cells collected. Healthcare Scientists should be aware that these cells may still be in store. The target (such as $>10 \times 10^8$/Kg nucleated cells), was calculated as a volume of the collection and the remainder discarded. These collections were often performed as an emergency for cellular depletion. The product was very concentrated with dilution and processing generally required immediately. It was important to check the volume of the product, which may be misrepresented by the apheresis machine due to the high blood viscosity.

14.3.9 Allogeneic Transplantation

Both bone marrow (HPC, Marrow) and peripheral blood stem cells (HPC, Apheresis) may be harvested from donors. These may be related or unrelated donors. It is imperative that documentation and products are labelled to enable reliable links. Prescribed target yields must be adjusted to the recipient's weight. Some unprocessed allogeneic harvests will require only quality monitoring, validation and labelling. These will then be issued for immediate reinfusion. Collections for registries such as the BBMR may be part of complex organisational chains involving couriers, international transport and international documentation. Healthcare Scientists may be involved in the receipt of cells imported from National or International registries. Local and registry protocols specifications and documentation must be familiar to technical staff. A 4°C hold may be required for HPC, Apheresis collections taking place on sequential days with international transport arranged when collections are complete. Communication may be required with a registry or transplant centre. Labelling may be quite different to local procedures and may involve anonymised donor or recipient identification. Technical staff need to be prepared and have access to the necessary protocols and personnel.

14.4 Accreditation and Regulation

Specific standards apply to the collection of HPC. FACT-JACIE Standards specify requirements for collection units, as they do for clinical and processing facilities. The Human Tissue Act specifies requirements for consent and for donation of allogeneic bone marrow and peripheral blood stem cells for transplantation, each within specific Codes of Practice. The World Marrow Donor Association specifies quality standards for unrelated Donor registries. All these standards are particularly concerned with the links between facilities, be they local or international. Healthcare Scientists should be aware of these specifications and any agreements relating to their facility.

14.5 Suggested Reading

1. FACT-JACIE International Standards for Cellular Therapy Product Collection, Processing and Administration (Current edition). www.jacie.org.

2. Department of Health Guidance on the Microbiological Safety of Human Organs, Tissues and Cells using Transplantation (2000). http://www.dh.gov.uk/en/Publicationsandstatistics/Publications/PublicationsPolicyAndGuidance/DH_4005526

3. BCSH Blood Transfusion Task Force. Guidelines for the collection, processing and storage of human bone marrow and peripheral blood stem cells for transplantation. Trans Med. 4: 165-172 (1994).

4. *Cellular Therapy. A Physician's Handbook.* Snyder EL, Haley NR (eds). Pages 11 - 32.

5. *Haemopoietic Stem Cell Transplantation. The EBMT Handbook.* Apperley J, Carreras E, Gluckman E, Gratwohl A, Masszi T (eds). Pages 79 – 106.

6. *Thomas' Hemopoietic Cell Transplantation.* Blume KG, Forman SJ, Applebaum FR (eds) Pages 538 – 549; 576 – 587.

7. Human Tissues Authority www.hta.gov.uk

14.6 Self Assessment Questions

Multiple Choice Questions

1. Stem cell donors must be mandatory tested for which of the following infectious agents:
   a) Hepatitis B
   b) HIV
   c) Hepatitis C
   d) Syphilis
   e) CMV

2. Which of the following parameters reflect the dose of stem cells on a HPC, Apheresis collection?
   a) number of CD133 cells
   b) number of CD34 cells
   c) number of CD3 cells
   d) TNC count
   e) RBC count

3. Bone marrow is usually harvested from which of the following sites?
   a) Posterior iliac crests
   b) Anterior iliac crests
   c) Femur
   d) Vertebrae
   e) Fibula

Short Answer Questions

1. Describe how stem cells are collected from peripheral blood by apheresis.

2. How are haematopoietic progenitor cells mobilised from the bone marrow? How is stem cell mobilisation monitored?

Assignments

1. Describe the special technical issues associated with the collection of stem cells from children. What does the HTA's Codes of Practice http://www.hta.gov.uk/ say about obtaining consent for such a procedure?

2. With reference to the latest FACT-JACIE standards www.jacie.org create a series of spider diagrams to describe a quality system intended to assure the safety and quality of stem cell collection activities.

15 PROCESSING AND QUALITY CONTROL OF HAEMATOPOIETIC STEM CELLS FOR TRANSPLANTATION

Note

This chapter refers to registered trade names and models from several manufacturers; there is no intention to endorse or recommend any particular device or manufacturer.

Processing may be defined as 'a series of actions which produce a change or development'. Clinical processing, in the context of stem cell transplantation, may be defined further as 'a modification of haematopoietic material which is desirable for a successful clinical outcome post transplant'. Processing normally involves the removal, enrichment or reduction of certain elements of the collection and commonly employs instrumentation specifically designed for cell separation/purification techniques. Procedures in use must be GMP-compliant. Processing may or may not be followed by cryopreservation of the cellular product before clinical use. Cryopreservation is covered in a separate chapter.

Expertise in cell separation and purification techniques needs to be accompanied by an understanding of haematopoiesis and cell biology. Knowledge of the immunology of transplantation and blood group serology is also essential as is an appreciation of the different mechanisms contributing to the success of autologous and allogeneic transplantation. A good understanding of the principles of physical separation techniques, monoclonal antibody based separation techniques including positive and negative selection is required.

15.1 Physical Separation Techniques

15.1.1 Plasma and Volume Reduction

This procedure is most commonly carried out for bone marrow collections (HPC, Marrow) where volumes collected can approach two litres. Plasma reduction would be required for allogeneic transplants where a minor ABO incompatibility exists between donor and recipient; a cell washing step may be included to further reduce the presence of donor plasma. Volume reduction is indicated for bone marrow collections prior to cryopreservation as volumes may be increased above clinically-acceptable levels by the addition of (an equivalent volume of) cryoprotectant. Reducing the volume of cryopreserved product also reduces the amount of cryoprotectant (dimethyl sulphoxide; DMSO) to which the patient will be exposed. Volume reduction also removes the majority of the red cells as these are haemolysed by the freezing/thawing process and can cause renal problems in the patient when infused.

These procedures are generally performed on an apheresis device such as the COBE 2991™. This device uses centrifugation combined with a single use sterile processing set. Variable centrifugation times and speeds allow separation of components while hydraulic fluid action against a flexible membrane expresses fluids or cells into a pre-attached waste or collection bag. Plasma and volume reduction of bone marrow on the COBE 2991™ results in a substantial reduction of red cell content as buffy coat is the final product. However, this level of depletion may not be sufficient in cases of major ABO incompatibility where almost complete depletion of red cells is required. In these cases the COBE Spectra™ may be used. HPC, Marrow up to 900ml can be processed using the COBE 2991™, larger volumes must be processed using the COBE Spectra.

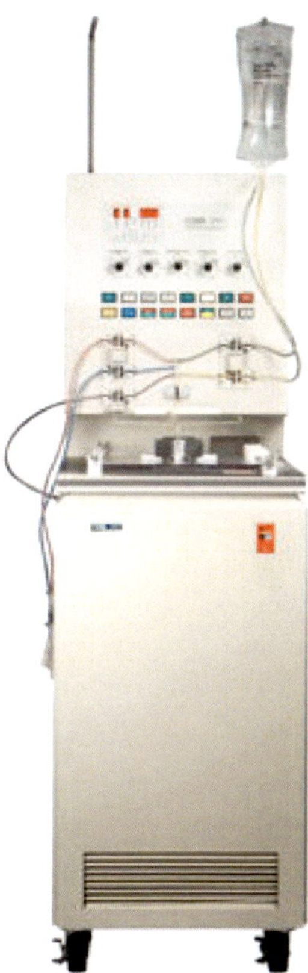

Figure 1 Cobe 2991 Device

15.1.2 Red Cell Depletion

As stated above this procedure is used in cases of major ABO incompatibility where almost complete depletion of red cells from allogeneic HPC, Marrow is required or when >900mls of HPC, Marrow is for processing. This may be achieved using the COBE Spectra™, an instrument which is very versatile and is the most popular for clinical apheresis procedures. The COBE Spectra™ is programmable and can be used for a number of procedures and like the COBE 2991™ it uses sterile processing sets. The COBE Spectra™ is more sophisticated than the 2991™ and although it too incorporates a centrifuge, it requires a greater level of expertise. During the procedure, anticoagulated HPC, Marrow enters the channel which is located in the centrifuge. As it flows through the channel, it is separated into three layers, the red cells on the outside, the buffy coat containing the white cells in the centre and the platelet rich plasma on the inside. The white cells are then collected through the WBC collect tube. Although the Spectra achieves volume reduction as part of its red cell depletion process it would not be the instrument of choice if simple centrifugation was adequate. Red cell depletion is not normally necessary from peripheral blood progenitor cell (HPC, Apheresis) collections.

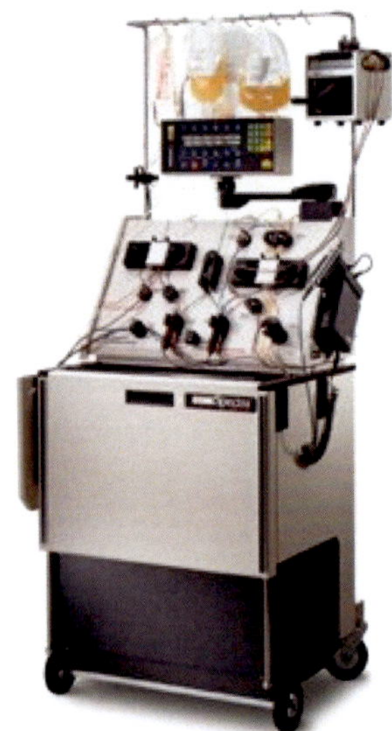

Figure 2. Cobe Spectra Device

15.1.3 Sepax

The Sepax is an automated closed processing system for blood and blood components with volumes between 35-800mls. The product is spun to create a centrifugal force that separates the components based on their density and size. It can be used to process HPC, Cord to isolate the buffy coat fraction. Hydroxy Ethyl Starch (HES) can be added to the system to allow a faster red cell sedimentation. The Sepax can also be used to volume reduce HPC, Apheresis and HPC, Marrow if required or to wash thawed products to remove DMSO.

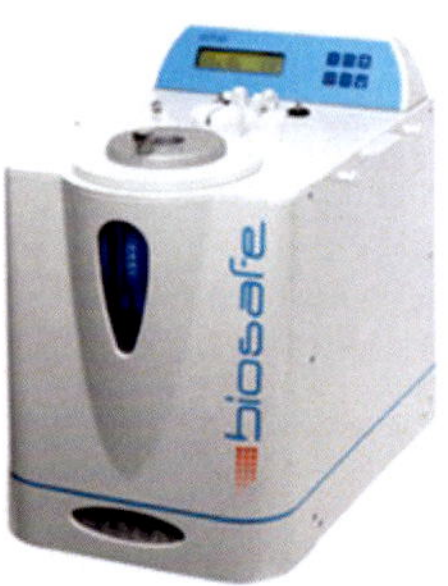

Figure 3 Sepax Device

15.1.4 Platelet Depletion

Platelets, like red cells, do not make a positive contribution to stem cell transplantation, but neither do they have an adverse affect on the graft *per se*. The high platelet numbers collected during a stem cell apheresis procedure may however cause problems if processing of a HPC, Apheresis collection is required, particularly after overnight storage when platelet clumping may be observed. Platelet depletion may be carried out by a low speed centrifugation / washing step on the COBE 2991™

15.2 Monoclonal Antibody-Based Techniques

Immunomagnetic cell separation systems can be used to select or deplete cell types for which specific monoclonal antibodies exist. An increasing portfolio of cell-specific monoclonal antibodies coupled to paramagnetic beads are available which may be used in conjunction with the Miltenyi CliniMACS for the clinical scale preparation of cells for specific therapies.

15.2.1 CD34 Selection

This procedure is carried out as a means of reducing the risk of GvHD following allogeneic transplant. It is a lengthy and costly procedure and is normally only carried out where there is a high degree of HLA mismatch between donor and patient (e.g. a haploidentical transplant). An alternative to CD34 selection is CD133 selection but the principal remains the same in that the cells that are required for transplant are 'positively' selected and retained separately from the negative fraction containing CD3+ve T cells which are implicated in the development of GvHD. T cell reduction to a predetermined dose per Kg patients body weight in the product is necessary and the Miltenyi CliniMACS™, an electro-mechanical device, is used for this procedure.

After a predetermined preparative procedure depending on the nature of the cellular harvest, monoclonal anti-CD34 antibody which is coupled to paramagnetic beads is added to the collection. Following incubation and washing, the bag containing the collection is connected to the CliniMACS set and passed through the system which incorporates a permanent magnet, a peristaltic pump and pinch valves. CD34$^+$ cells bound by antibody to the magnetic beads are retained by the magnet allowing the T cell rich fraction to pass into a collection bag. Following washing of the retained cells, CD34$^+$ cells are eluted from the magnet into a separate product bag. The CliniMACS™ is capable of 4-5 log depletion of T cells in the product compared to the starting material. The T cell 'waste' fraction may be used to add a small dose of T cells back to the product if deemed appropriate to aid engraftment or for cryopreservation as aliquots of donor lymphocytes (DLI) for post transplant therapy.

Negative selection procedures may also be carried out on the CliniMACS™ using the same principle. Where CD3 depletion is required (as above) monoclonal antibody to CD3 would be employed to extract CD3$^+$ T cells from the harvest leaving CD34$^+$ cells and accessory cells, depleted of T cells available for transplant.

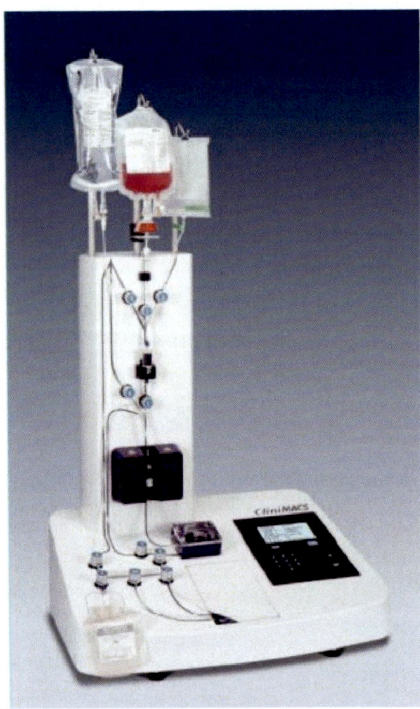

Figure 4. CliniMacs Device

15.2.2 CD3/CD19 Depletion.

This represents a different approach to minimising GvHD post-transplant. CD34$^+$ cell selection has been successful in permitting the transplantation of grafts between haplo-identical donors and recipients, typically from parent and child and ideally using CD34$^+$ cell doses of greater than 20 x 10^6/kg. Graft failures still occur however, and the most common cause in this context is relapse as a result of the profound T cell depletion afforded by CD34$^+$ cell selection. A certain minimum number of CD3$^+$ cells of the order of 1 - 5x 10^4/Kg has been shown to be beneficial in promoting engraftment and now other cells in a cellular harvest are recognised as contributing to patient recovery and survival. These are NK cells, T- cell progenitors, monocytes and dendritic cells and so-called 'facilitating cells'. Thus the selective removal of CD3$^+$ T cells from a harvest together with CD19$^+$ B lymphocytes which are implicated in the development of EBV-mediated post transplant lymphoproliferative disease is seen as having considerable benefits over CD34$^+$ cell selection. Data from clinical trials suggest this alternative approach results in a faster recovery of platelets, an enhanced GvL effect due to the cytotoxic effect of NK cells against leukaemic cells, faster immune recovery and a reduced incidence of viral infections post transplant.

From a laboratory perspective the procedure takes longer to complete than CD34$^+$ cell selection:

1. Accurate percentages of labelled cells, assayed immediately pre-selection, total nucleated cell concentration need to be programmed into the CliniMACS™ as well as total cell volume to be processed. This is in contrast to CD34 selection which has no requirement for data entry.

2. Higher numbers of cells labelled with antibody have to be captured by the CliniMACS™ magnet. Loading is staged to deal with this effectively and as a result the procedure takes more time.

3. Flow cytometry is more extensive and time consuming as several cell populations which might, incorrectly, be included in a T cell count need to be excluded. More significantly, T cell numbers remaining in the product should be rare events and for a statistically significant T cell assay as many as 750,000 events may have to be counted.

15.2.3 NK Cell Selection

NK (CD56$^+$) cells may be prepared for adoptive immunotherapy as an alternative to DLI. As discussed above they have potent anti-tumour activity but unlike DLI do not have the disadvantage of contributing to GvHD. They may even reduce the risk of GVHD by targeting KIR mismatched antigen-presenting cells (APCs) of the recipient. CD3$^+$ cell depletion prior to positive CD56$^+$ cell selection provides a highly enriched NK cell fraction.

15.2.4 Use of Campath 'in the bag'

Campath-1H is a humanised IgG1 monoclonal antibody directed against the CD52 antigen on human lymphocytes. It can be added to a bag of HPC prior to infusion in the patient to deplete T cells from the product.

15.3 Quality Control

For stem cell products it is important to have accurate methods for counting the number of cells. The methods available vary from manual and subjective to fully automated and quantitative. The need for accurate cell counting is several fold and includes:

- TNC count – important prior to addition of cryoprotectant;

- Total CD3 count – important prior to and after T cell reduction;

- Total CD34 count – important during stem cell mobilisation and after collection to determine available of stem cells for transplantation.

In addition to the total cell counts listed above it is also important to have an indication of the viability/ growth potential of the stem cell product as this will assess the potential of the product for engraftment.

15.3.1 Marrow and Blood Smears

This is one of the simplest methods of determining the white cell differential in a sample. Firstly, the white cell count needs to be obtained. This is most easily done using a counting chamber. The sample is diluted in a fluid that contains acetic acid to lyse the red cells and a dye such as gentian violet that stains the white cells. To obtain the white cell differential a small drop of the sample if placed on a glass slide and is smeared using a second slide. The smear is air dried and fixed in methanol. The smears are then stained using for example Wright's or Leishman's stain; these contain eosin and methylene blue. The relative percentages of the different cell types in the smear are obtained by counting a minimum of 200 consecutive nucleated cells.

15.3.2 Haematology Analysers

Haematology analysers are multifunctional instruments that can not only provide the user with the total white cell count including the differential but can also give counts for platelet and red cell concentration together with a measure of the haemoglobin content, haematocrit and mean cell volume. The analyser draws up a sample of blood passing this through a narrow tubing and using various sensors counts the cells. The two main sensors being light detection and electrical impedance.

Modern haematology analysers' use various methods to obtain the differential cell count but are all based on using differential lysing solutions together with granular stains. After treatment in the respective solutions, the cells are passed by the detectors. The different white cells each have their own unique nuclear and morphological structure and because of this absorb light differently. The signals from the light absorbance and the changes in impedance (a change in resistance is proportional to the volume of the cell) are correlated and combined by electronic processing to define the white cell differential. Because the analyser can count large numbers of cells over a relatively short period of time it can give a very precise estimate of the cell numbers.

15.3.3 Flow Cytometry

Similar to the haematology analyser the flow cytometer analyses cells populations by exposing them to a beam of light and detecting the resulting light scatter. The cells are exposed to the light source after undergoing a process of hydrodynamic focussing whereby a single stream of cells is produced. In flow cytometry, the cells are normally labelled most commonly with antibodies that detect a surface antigen of particular interest. The antibodies are conjugated to a fluorescent dye which, when stimulated by light of a particular wavelength, will emit light of a different wavelength. This light is then focussed onto a light detector and a signal generated. From the combination of different antibodies, dyes, optical filters and multiple detectors together with a complex computational analysis, a picture of the different cell populations within a sample is obtained. By adding a specific volume of calibrated beads to the sample prior to analysis an absolute count of the cells within the sample can be determined (single platform). Alternatively, the percentage differential of the cell populations in the sample can be determined together with the white cell count from a basic haematology analyser an absolute cell count can be determined (dual platform). However, the single platform system has been found by quality assurance schemes to be the most accurate for absolute cell counting.

For stem cell collections, CD34 cell enumeration has become the most widely used for measuring the stem and progenitor cell content. The CD34 antigen is a monomeric transmembrane phosphoglycoprotein of about 110Kda, the extracellular portion of which contains two distinct domains. The CD34 antigen is expressed on haematopoietic progenitor cells of all lineages. Its expression is highest on the most primitive of stem cells and is gradually lost as lineage committed progenitors differentiate. A number of CD34 antibodies have been described that detect the three broad classes of epitopes expressed on some or all of the CD34 glycoforms. For enumeration of CD34 cells in mobilised peripheral blood and apheresis products, phycoeythrin conjugated antibodies to either the Class II or III epitopes are preferred.

There are several flow cytometric analytical protocols described for CD34 cell quantitation but the one most commonly used is that known as the 'ISHAGE protocol'. This protocol uses dual staining with fluorescein isothiocyanate (FITC)-conjugated anti-CD45 antibodies and phycoerythrin (PE)-conjugated anti-CD34 antibodies. Sequential gating first with CD45-positive cells, then with CD34-positive/low side scatter cells followed by back gating to CD45 with side scatter ensures selection of the true CD34 stem cell population.

The addition of 7-aminoactinomycin D (7-AAD) to the sample prior to analysis means an estimate of the cell viability can be obtained. This is not however a true estimate of viability as it is only a measurement of membrane integrity which is associated with cell viability.

Figure 5 Principles of flow cytometry

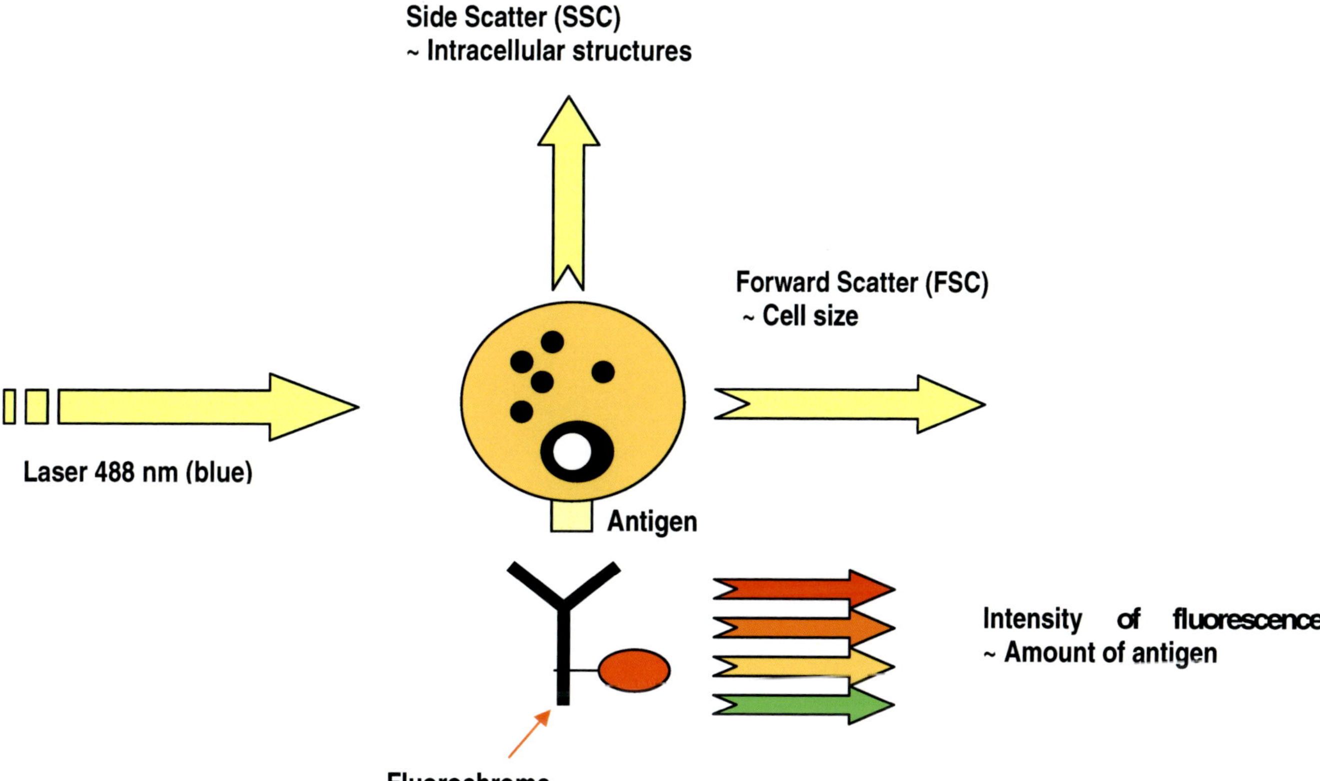

Figure 6 ISHAGE Gating Protocol

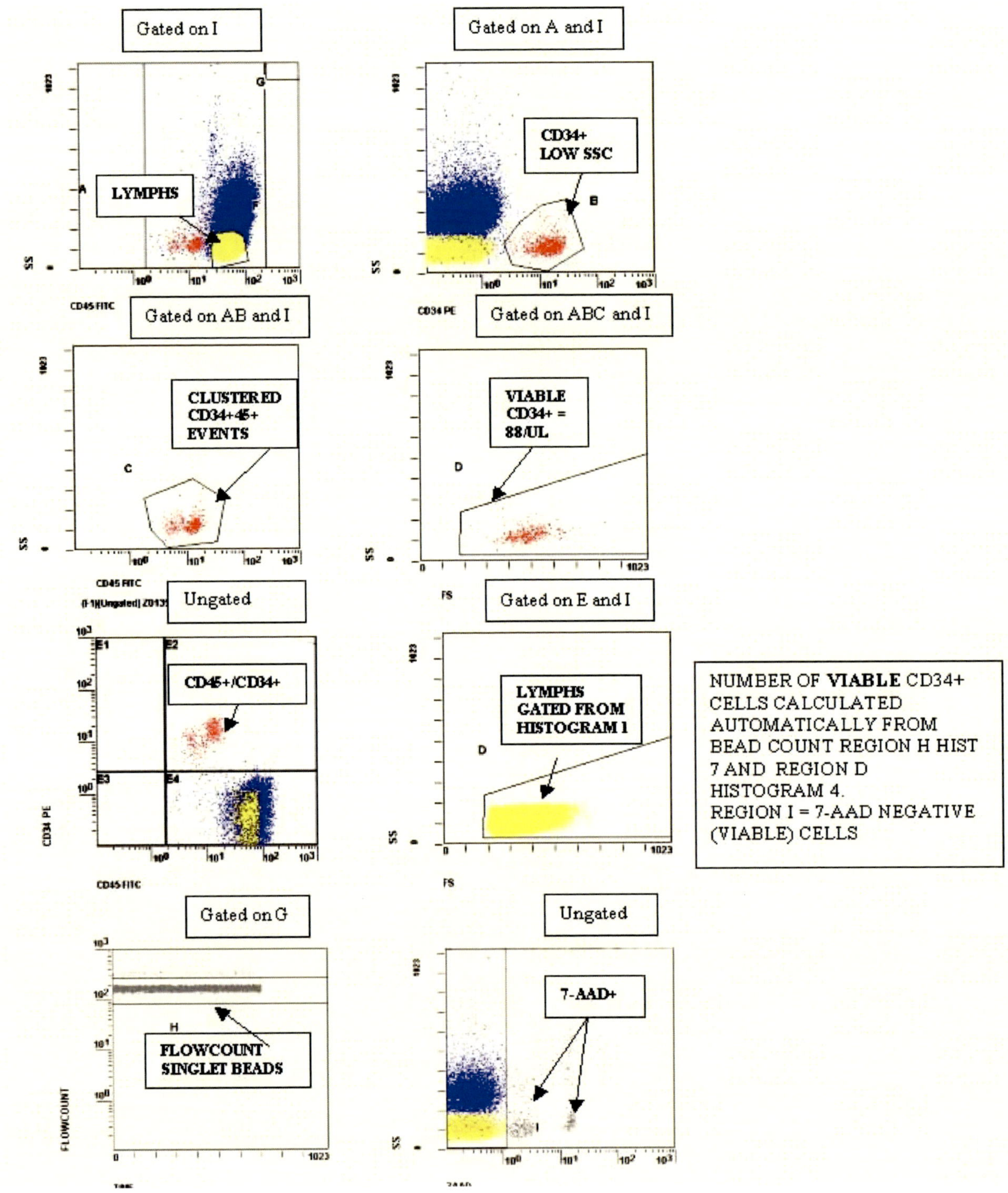

15.3.4 Cell Culture Assays

Although flow cytometric analysis of cell populations can give an accurate estimate of cell number and viability it does not reflect the ability of the cells to proliferate. *In vitro* culture assays have been developed to detect the proliferation and differentiation ability of haematopoietic cells. The most common approach to quantify progenitor cells utilises viscous or semi solid media together with supplements that permit the proliferation and differentiation of the cells whilst allowing the development of discrete visible cell colonies. Culture media have been optimised for growth of erythroid, monocyte/macrophage, granulocytic, megakaryocytic and multipotent progenitor cells. An important aspect of haematopoietic cell culture is the standardisation of the culture conditions, not only the culture medium but also the temperature; humidity, O_2 and CO_2 levels plus the incubation time before colonies are scored. Furthermore the method used to prepare the cells, their purity; concentration and the mixture of growth factors can also influence the results obtained.

Clonogenic progenitors of granulocytes (CFU-G), macrophages (CFU-M), or both (CFU-GM) are defined on their ability to produce colonies with a minimum of 20 or 50 of these cells. Two different types of media can be used to generate granulopoietic colonies. These are both methylcellulose-based differing by the addition of recombinant growth factors or agar and leukocyte-conditioned media (LCM). Methylcellulose media containing LCM can be used to assay for both erythroid and granulopoietic precursors in the same culture. When this is the case it is recommended to maintain cells in culture for least 18 days and for plates to be examined on a regular basis from 10 days onwards before scoring the cultures to avoid wrongly scoring the early stage erythroid colonies as granulocyte and macrophage colonies. When the methylcellulose media contains recombinant growth factors a larger proportion of the granulopoietic colonies will achieve a larger size than in medium containing LCM.

Figure 7 Cell colony types identified in CFU assays

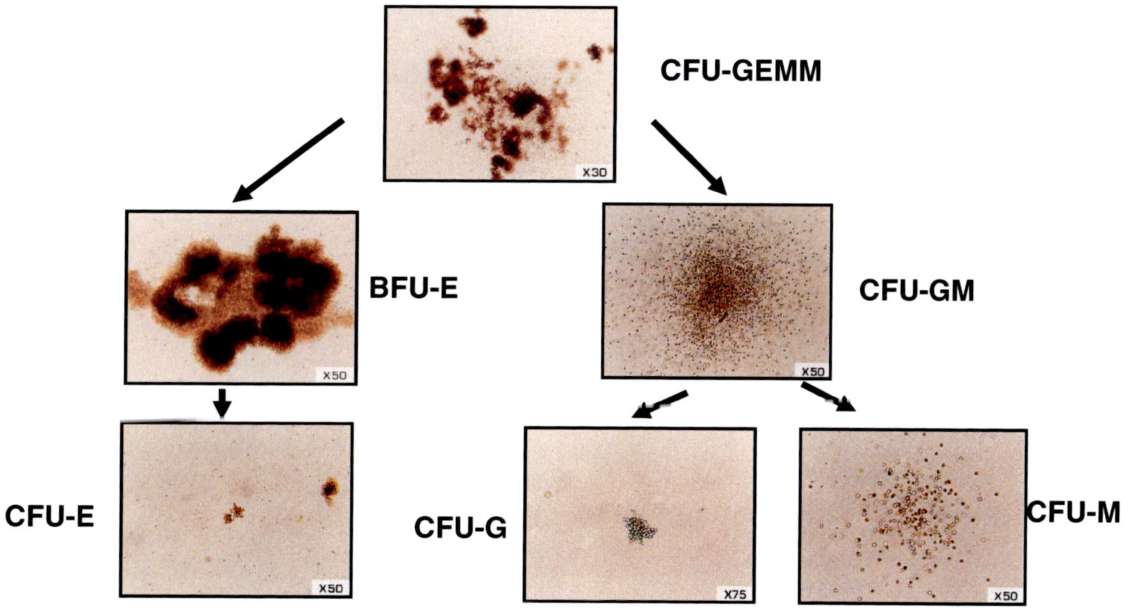

In general a value of 2×10^4 CFU-GM/Kg body weight is predictive of cell engraftment. In comparison the threshold for engraftment based on CD34 count is 2×10^6/Kg; below this level the likelihood of delayed engraftment increases.

15.4 Suggested Reading

1. *Bone Marrow and Stem Cell Processing: A Manual of Current Techniques.* Areman EM, Deeg HJ, Sacher RA (eds). F.A. Davis. Philadelphia

2. *Cellular Therapy. A Physicians Handbook.* Snyder EL, Haley NR (eds). Pages 51 to 79

3. Information on COBE 2991™ and COBE Spectra™.
   http://www.caridianbct.com/location/emea/Pages/home.aspx

4. Information on the Cytomate™ and CliniMACS™ devices. www.miltenyibiotec.com/

5. Iyengar R *et al.* (2003) Purification of human natural killer cells using a clinical scale immunomagnetic method. Cytotherapy, 5:479-484

6. Ruggeri L *et al.* (1999) Role of natural killer cell alloreactivity in HLA-mismatched hematopoietic stem cell transplantation. Blood, 94:333-339

7. Introduction to flow cytometry
   http://probes.invitrogen.com/resources/education/tutorials/4Intro_Flow/player.html

15.5 Self Assessment Questions

Multiple Choice Questions

1. Which of the following markers characterise a haematopoietic stem cell?
    a) CD32
    b) CD133
    c) CD34
    d) CD3
    e) CD43

2. A COBE Spectra™ can be used for which of the following manipulations?
    a) Red cell depletion
    b) CD34 cell selection
    c) CD34 cell depletion
    d) Plasma depletion
    e) Leucodepletion

3. Which of the following statements are true of CD34 cells which are <u>not</u> stained by 7-AAD?
    a) The cells are viable
    b) The cells will engraft
    c) The cells are dead
    d) The cells have a membrane capable of excluding the dye
    e) The cells are relatively primitive stem cells

4. Which of the following statements are true? Depletion of CD3 cells is important to:
    a) Increase the rate to engraftment
    b) Increase the GvL effect
    c) Reduce GvHD
    d) Allow haplo-identical transplants
    e) Reduce DMSO toxicity.

Short Answer Questions

2. Describe the operation of a sterile connecting device

3. Explain the principle of CD34 cell selection using the CliniMACS.

Assignments

1. In an effort to reduce the amount of time staff are spending in clean rooms, your manager has asked you to consider the feasibility of performing bone marrow processing on a COBE Spectra™ in an 'unclassified' laboratory. Prepare a short feasibility study including a risk assessment and recommendations.

2. Prepare a specification for a flow cytometer which a stem cell laboratory might use for quality control of stem cell products.

16 CORD BLOOD BANKING

16.1 Introduction

Cord blood (CB) provides a source of haematopoietic stem cells used as a therapeutic option in the bone marrow transplantation setting. CB was identified as an alternate source of stem cells when the first CB transplant between siblings, for Fanconi's anaemia, in 1989 led to a successful outcome. The first unrelated CB bank (CBB) was established in New York in 1993 followed shortly by the development of banks in most major countries, with the objective to collect and store large panels of CB units providing a broad range of HLA types.

CB is the blood that remains in the placenta and umbilical cord after the birth of the baby. CB can be collected, tested, cryopreserved and stored for years without the loss of potency of the stem cells, providing an 'on the shelf' product that can be made available for use in the clinic within a few days.

About one third of patients requiring a bone marrow (BM) transplant find a match within their own family, for the remainder a search is performed of the bone marrow registries. Unfortunately many patients are unable to undergo BM transplantation because of the lack of a suitable donor or because their disease cannot wait for the time required to find and prepare a matched BM donor. In practice, many patients, particularly those from the ethnic minorities, cannot find a suitable match. CB offers a viable option for these patients.

16.2 Advantages of Cord Blood Banking

Historically, cord blood has been used predominantly for transplantation in children due to concerns that the low cell 'dose' might make it less suitable for patients with a larger body mass. For paediatric patients, cord is regarded as a readily accessible stem cell source which may achieve less GvHD, improved T-cell reconstitution (Chiesa et al. In press) and improved graft versus leukaemia (GvL) effect (Eapen et al. 2007; Wagner et al. 2009). A review of clinical outcomes following CBT in children concluded that, in the absence of a matched sibling, transplant outcomes for cord blood were comparable and possibly superior to bone marrow, depending on the circumstances. Though for bone marrow failure, matched bone marrow is still preferable as a source for children with acute leukaemia cord blood may be equivalent or even superior (Hough et al. 2009). A recent study found that 5-year leukaemia-free survival for paediatric patients transplanted with 1 or 2 antigen mismatched cord blood was comparable to using matched bone marrow, while matched cord blood appeared to achieve better results (Eapen et al. 2007). A meta-analysis of recent outcome studies with unrelated bone marrow transplants (BMTs) and cord blood transplants (CBTs) concluded that unrelated CBT in children and adults had consistently equivalent survival outcomes compared with unrelated BMT despite greater donor-recipient HLA disparity with unrelated CBT (Hwang et al. 2007).

In the adult setting, it has recently become clear that by selecting cord blood units containing high doses of stem cells and through the use of two units, good outcomes can also be obtained in patients with a higher body mass. In 2004, two major studies, performed by Eurocord and the Center for International Bone Marrow Transplant Research (CIBMTR), reported similar outcomes for CBT when compared to unrelated HSCT using BM or PBSC. These studies concluded that, in the absence of a matched unrelated adult donor, matched or mismatched cord blood was an acceptable stem cell source (Laughlin et al. 2004; Rocha et al. 2004). Subsequently, interest in the therapeutic potential of CBT in adults has intensified as a clearer picture of its clinical potential has developed.

The advantages of cord blood may be summarised as follows:

- CB is abundantly and readily available, with the collection posing no risk to the donor.
- Ethnic minority groups are markedly under represented in BM registries. By targeting collection in areas where the obstetric population is diverse, a wide spectrum of ethnic donations and hence HLA types can be harvested.
- CB requires less stringent HLA matching between the donor and recipient than is required for BM donors. This means that the efficacy of finding a match in a CBB is higher than from a BM registry.
- A unit of CB from the bank can be identified and made available for transplantation within days, reducing the morbidity and death in patients associated with the longer procurement times for BM. This is of particular benefit for patients with a rapidly progressing malignant disease.
- CB has a lower incidence of viral infection than found in adult BM donors, particularly for cytomegalovirus (CMV), which can cause profound illness in BM transplantation patients.
- A lower incidence of graft-versus-host disease (GvHD) is reported in CB transplantation for both children and adults, contributing to reduced morbidity compared with BM transplantation.

16.3 Disadvantages of Cord Blood Banking

The disadvantages of cord blood may be summarised as follows:

- BM donors may be recalled for the same recipient to provide either a second donation of BM or a donation of lymphocytes to provide passive immunity for a variety of disorders. However, CB donations are of limited size and it is not ethical to seek additional donations from the neonatal donor.
- BM donors can provide a medical history at the time of donation that is relevant to the donation. However, CB donors provide the medical history through their mothers and because CB can be stored for decades, future disorders in the donor may not be apparent at the time of donation. Examples of a genetic disorder not apparent at the time of birth are sickle cell disease or a metabolic syndrome. These risks are minimised by stringent donor selection and testing where appropriate. Mothers are invited to report the development of relevant illnesses in due course.

16.4 Categories of Cord Blood Banking

CB may be collected and banked for altruistic unrelated use or be banked for family use either for an existing sick child or for 'insurance purposes' in the future. The use of autologous blood is rare.

16.4.1 Directed Donations

If a family has a child with a disorder which could be treated by BM transplantation or its equivalent, then the clinician looking after the sick child may request a directed CB donation from any subsequent healthy child of the same parents. The chances of an HLA match are one in four for children of the same parents and the chances of a recessive genetic disease being present are also one in four. Pre-implantation diagnosis for genetic disease and for screening for tissue type can theoretically be undertaken, but in practice, the chances of a matching sibling having the genetic disease are only 1 in 16.

An additional category of directed banking relates to the commercial sector. Families who do not have a family member with a disease needing a BMT sometimes request directed donations. The CB is collected and reserved only for their family use. NHSBT does not undertake this type of banking - in the UK it is performed by commercial organisations. Companies invite individual families to store CB at the time of delivery of a normal child for 'insurance purposes'. Information on these commercial companies is widely available in literature provided to women in the antenatal period and is also available on numerous web sites. The UK Royal College of Obstetricians has issued guidance relating to this type of banking.

An argument against autologous transplantation of CB relates to the lack of graft versus leukaemia (GvL) effect and the demonstration that leukaemic cells or genetic markers of disease may be present in the fetal blood of patients before a disease is diagnosed.

16.4.2 Unrelated Donations

For unrelated banking, CB is collected from volunteer donors in selected hospitals that have maternity units with a high rate of normal deliveries and a diverse ethnic mix. Unrelated donations are made available for patients world-wide.

16.5 Regulation of Cord Blood Banks

CB banking operates in a highly regulated environment. Currently regulated by the Human Tissue Authority (HTA) in the UK and by FACT-NETCORD internationally. The Food and Drug Administration (FDA) in the USA have regulations for good tissue practice, that became effective in May 2005, and the EU adopted a Directive for Tissues and Cells in 2004, to which member states needed to comply from 2006. Standards for CB banking cover all aspects from collection, processing, testing, banking, selection and release.

Unrelated CB banking is conducted in a number of different ways at different banks, involving many steps in the process. Figure 1 details the operational process at the NHS Cord Blood Bank.

16.6 Donor Recruitment

Recruitment of donors, consent and donor selection and testing are all functions related to the practice of CB banking and all are subject to a variety of ethical issues. For maternal donor's genuine informed consent to be given for a variety of activities, full information must be provided to the potential donor mothers so that an informed choice about whether to donate to the unrelated CBB can be made, particularly where there are commercial CB banking enterprises available. This means that when donors are recruited, information must be provided in an easily accessible way that the donors can understand – leaflets, posters and presentations. At an interview with the mother the formal aspects of participation in CB banking are discussed. Explanations are given as to the purpose of CB banking, the life saving potential of CB, the benefits and alternatives, such as commercial banking, and the right of the mother to refuse to donate without prejudice to her or her baby's care. Ethnic background information is obtained to provide data for the transplant centre to help them in making an informed choice of which unit to select for transplant.

16.6.1 Consent

Consent includes donation, maternal and CB testing, and use of the donation. The consent procedure covers a variety of clauses as shown in Table 1, that have developed to address the ethical issues in collecting CB and legal requirements. Consent must not be obtained while the mother is in active labour or under anaesthesia.

16.6.2 Donor Selection

Donor information is required to ensure the safety and appropriateness of a donation for a potential recipient. A medical risk assessment, following a standard questionnaire, includes a review of behavioural risks for HIV and hepatitis B and C, skin piercing, blood transfusion, including the presence of transmissible infections. Travel history, medical and genetic background of the donor parents helps reduce the risk of transmissible diseases and predisposition to disorders or genetic diseases. At the NHS CBB the mother is telephoned post natally to check on her health and her baby's.

16.7 Cord Blood Collection

The objective of the collection procedure is to maximise the volume of CB harvested from the placenta whilst reducing the risks of contamination from bacteria, fungi, maternal blood and secretions, without influencing or interfering with the routine delivery procedures. CB can be collected from the placenta following normal vaginal delivery or caesarean section by either *in utero* or *ex utero* methods.

16.7.1 In Utero

A trained member of the delivery team can collect the blood in the delivery room during the third stage of labour while the placenta is still *in utero*. To perform *in utero* collection, consent for collection must be obtained prior to delivery. *In utero* collection avoids the possibility of a failed collection due to damage to the placenta but may pose potential conflicts of interest for the staff caring for the mother and baby.

16.7.2 Ex Utero

Alternatively, collection can be performed *ex utero* in an adjacent room after delivery of the placenta by trained delivery or CBB staff. The use of a small number of dedicated staff facilitates management of staff training and reduces variability in the collection procedure.

Following robust cleaning of the umbilical cord, a prominent umbilical cord vessel is selected, a needle is inserted and the blood flows through the needle into the collection bag under gravity. Acceptable values for volume and cell content of the units are established to ensure that the collection meets the requirements of the transplant centres.

16.8 Cord Blood Processing

A successful CB bank requires long-term storage of a large number of units. This introduces space issues that have been addressed by reducing the volume of CB unit prior to storage. A number of methods are in use, the majority of which deplete the unit of red cells and plasma in a closed system, leaving the stem cells in a standard volume, whilst maintaining the quality and quantity of the stem cells. Dedicated equipment is now also available for CB processing. Use of the 'waste' plasma and red cells for testing and archiving, permits the bank to maximise the storage of the collected stem cells. Samples are removed from the CB unit throughout the process for testing, quality monitoring and archiving, for future testing at issue for transplant.

To preserve the cells they are cryopreserved in 10% DMSO and stored in liquid nitrogen at temperatures below −150°C, giving an average of 80% recovery of nucleated cells (NC) and >90% recovery of CD34+ cells.

16.9 Cord Blood Testing

16.9.1 Microbiology

Both the donor mother and CB unit are tested to ensure safety for the transplant patient. Testing of the mother and CB for infectious diseases is the same as that for blood donors, and includes tests for HIV, hepatitis B and C, syphilis and HTLV. More sensitive nucleic acid tests (NAT) of the mother for HIV, HBV and HCV are required at banking of the CB unit. If these tests are not available a further sample from the mother taken at 180 days post delivery is used to exclude infections in the 'window period' at the time of delivery. A wider array of tests are performed when a CB unit is selected for transplant. A sample of CB from the final product, prior to cryopreservation, is screened for bacterial and fungal contamination.

16.9.2 Haematology

A full blood count (FBC) is performed on a pre-process sample of the CB unit to assess the normality of the baby and to calculate the total nucleated cell content of the donation. Post-process the FBC is repeated as a quality measure of the process, and as an indicator of the CB unit engraftment potential. Only units that contain sufficient cells for transplantation are accepted into the bank. Review of the blood film provides a nucleated red cell count and an indication of infection or a congenital abnormality such as spherocytosis. At issue for transplantation an expert in neonatal haematology reviews the blood film.

16.9.3 Tissue Typing

All CB units are tissue typed, as are BM donors. It is this tissue type that is used to select the CB unit or BM donor that will provide a suitable match for the patient requiring a BM transplant. Some tissue types are more common in particular ethnic backgrounds, therefore in addition to matching a CB donation and patient's tissue type it is also important to consider the ethnic background.

The minimum requirements are for the units to be typed for HLA-A, B & DR. At the time the unit is reserved for transplant confirmatory tissue typing and high resolution typing are performed. The maternal archive sample is HLA typed to confirm the linkage to the CB donation.

16.9.4 Stem Cells

Counting the number of CD34+ cells assesses the stem cell content of the CB unit. CD34+ cell content and viability are performed by flow cytometry, on a sample from the final product, prior to cryopreservation. At the time of issue a sample of the cryopreserved unit is assayed for its functional, proliferative ability using a colony-forming assay and the CD34+ cell recovery is determined.

     128

16.10 Registration of Cord Blood Units

On completion of processing, testing and interview a medical officer reviews the donor and donation information for suitability of the unit for inclusion into the bank. Prior to release for search a quality check is performed on each donation to ensure compliance with standards and specifications.

On release of the donation the units are made available for search through registration with national and international BM and CB registries. The units are registered under a unique identifier and the following data is provided: HLA type, volume of collected CB and total nucleated cell count of the final product.

16.11 Search, Issue and Release for Transplantation

Transplant centres initiate a search for CB units in the same way as for BM donors. Most BM donor registries hold both BM and CB information so that a search request can provide a comprehensive list of compatible donors/donations. Once a transplant centre receives a match report direct contact is made with the relevant CBB. There are a number of steps involved in the selection and release of a unit for transplantation and CB banks vary in how this is managed – an example from the NHS CBB is provided in Table 2.

Units are selected on both their tissue type and nucleated cell dose. It is widely accepted and recommended by Eurocord that a CB unit should provide a minimum pre-freeze nucleated cell dose of 2.0×10^7/kg patient body weight and at least a 4/6 HLA match. Once transplanted follow up data is obtained from the transplant centre as the final quality measure of the process of the CBB.

Following analysis of the outcome data from increasing numbers of CB transplants improved criteria for selecting appropriate matched units is slowly emerging. As of 2006 the following recommendations were made by Eurocord:

Patients with malignant diseases:

- Cell dose is the most important factor for outcome - a minimum of 3×10^7 TNC/kg patient body weight at collection or 2×10^7 TNC/kg at infusion.
- HLA mismatches increase the risk of delayed engraftment, transplant related mortality and cGVHD
- Increasing the cell dose abrogates the effect of HLA mismatches

Patients with non-malignant diseases:

- A minimum of 4.9×10^7 TNC/kg patient body weight at collection or 3.5×10^7 TNC/kg at infusion.
- HLA mismatches play a major role in engraftment, GvHD and survival
- Increasing cell dose only partially abrogates the effect of HLA mismatches

Figure 1. Cord Blood Banking Process at the NHSBT Cord Blood Bank

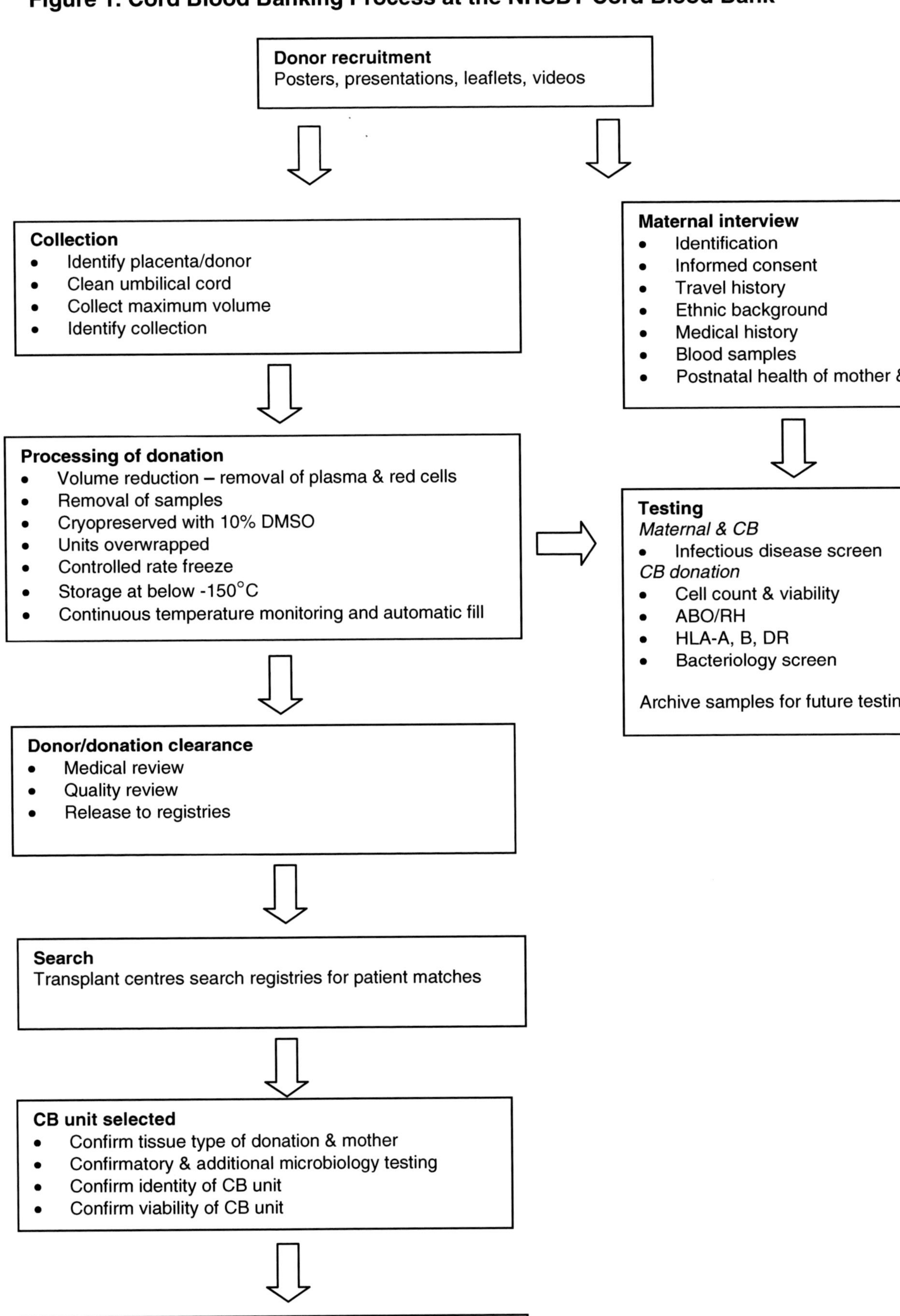

Table 1. Consent for Cord Blood Banking

Activities Requiring Consent
Collection and storage of CB for transplantation into unrelated individuals in the UK and abroad
Examination of the mother's and infant's relevant medical notes and dialogue with relevant clinical professionals
Permission for microbiological testing, including for HIV, and for the donor to be counselled in the event of results relevant to their health
Storage of samples for future testing, including new infections that may emerge in the future
Storage of personal information
Exchange of information relating to the donation with CB/BM Registries and transplant centres world-wide
Research and development use if the donation is unsuitable for clinical use

Table 2. Search, Issue & Release for Transplantation

Activity	Detail
Search	Transplant Centre initiates search of registries for patient match.
TC contacts CBB	
CBB provides a preliminary report	• Degree of HLA compatibility; • Volume of CB collection pre & post process; • Cell content; • Microbiology status of mother; • Bacteriology status of CB unit; • Ethnic background; • Donor sex.
Potential selection of CB unit – transplant centre reserves unit, CBB performs confirmatory & additional tissue type testing	• Confirmatory & high resolution HLA typing of CB unit; • Maternal HLA typing; • Mandatory microbiology screening of CB; • CMV NAT on CB; • Confirmatory microbiology testing with increased sensitivity & wider range of organisms; • Blood film examined by paediatric haematologist; • Clinical summary.
TC confirms selection, CBB confirms identity and viability of unit	• Short tandem repeat (STR) analysis performed on bleedline segment from unit in parallel with original CB sample • Colony forming unit (CFU) analysis on thawed sample • TC provide sample from patient • CB bank provides DNA sample from unit
Issue	• Shipping arrangements • Handling instructions
Transplant	• TC provide CB bank with follow-up data

Key
CB; cord blood
CFU: colony forming unit
CMV; cytomegalovirus
TC; transplant centre
STR; short tandem repeat analysis

16.12 Suggested Reading

1. Armitage S. Collection and Processing of Cord Blood Units. In: *Cord Blood Characteristics: Role in Stem Cell Transplantation*. Eds SBA Cohen, E Gluckman, P Rubinstein, JA Madrigal. Dunitz. Pp 129-148 (1999).

2. Gluckman E. Editorial: Hematopoietic stem cell transplants using UCB. N Engl J Med. 344:1860-1861 (2001).

3. Chiesa M. et al. Umbilical cord blood transplantation without serotherapy in children is associated with rapid CD4+ reconstitution t-cell reconstitution and recovery of anti-viral responses. Abstract. (2010).

4. Eapen M. et al. Outcomes of transplantation of unrelated donor umbilical cord blood and bone marrow in children with acute leukaemia: a comparison study. Lancet, 369 (9577), 1947-54 (2007).

5. Hough R. et al. Allogeneic haemopoietic stem cell transplantation in children: what donor should we choose when no matched sibling is available? British Journal of Haematology, 147(5): 593-613 (2009).

6. Hwang WY. et al. A meta-analysis of unrelated donor umbilical cord blood transplantation versus unrelated donor bone marrow transplantation in adult and paediatric patients. Biology of Blood and Marrow Transplantation, 13(4): 444-53 (2007).

7. Laughlin MJ. et al. Hematopoietic engraftment and survival in adult recipients of umbilical cord blood from unrelated donors. N Engl J Med. 344: 1815-1822 (2001).

8. Laughlin MJ. et al. Outcomes after transplantation of cord blood or bone marrow from unrelated donors in adults with leukaemia. The New England Journal of Medicine, 351(22): 2265-75 (2004).

9. Rocha V. et al. Comparison of outcomes of unrelated BM and UCB transplants in children with acute leukemia. Blood, 97: 2962-2971 (2001).

10. Sugarman J. et al. Consensus statement: ethical issues in umbilical cord blood banking. JAMA. 278: 938-943 (1997).

11. Wagner J. Should double cord transplants be the preferred choice when a sibling donor is unavailable? Best Pract Res Clin Haematol, 22(4): 551-5 (2009).

12. Scientific Advisory Committee for the Royal Colleges of Obstetricians and Gynaecologists. Umbilical cord blood banking. SAC Opinion paper 2; revised June 2006. [http://www.rcog.org.uk/index.asp?PageID=545]

13. Broxmeyer, HE. Biology of cord blood cells and future prospects for enhanced clinical benefit. Cytotherapy, 7:209-218 (2005).

14. On Line Cord Blood Forum. http://www.cordbloodforum.org

16.13 Self Assessment Questions

Multiple Choice Questions

1. Which of the following deliveries would be suitable for collection of cord blood for banking?
   a) Over 34 weeks gestation
   b) Under 34 weeks gestation
   c) Over 40 weeks gestation
   d) Over 36 weeks gestation
   e) Over 38 weeks gestation

2. Which of the following should be worn when collecting cord blood?
   a) Face mask
   b) Plastic apron
   c) Theatre shoes
   d) Non latex gloves
   e) Theatre suit

3. Which of the following combinations is sufficient to identify a donor mother?
   a) First name + surname
   b) First name + surname + date of birth
   c) Full name + address
   d) Full name + date of birth
   e) Full name + address + date of birth

4. Which criteria are used for deciding if a cord blood unit is acceptable for processing?
   a) Volume is over 40mL
   b) Total nucleated cell count is over $40 \times 10^7/mL$
   c) Less than 2 hours since collection
   d) No large clots
   e) Collection and paper work correctly labelled

Short Answer Questions

1. The aim of the cord blood collection procedure is to maximise the volume collected. Why is this important?

2. If the donor mother states that they have been abroad in the last year, what information needs to be taken? Why is this information important?

Assignments

1. Discuss the pros and cons of *in utero* versus *ex utero* cord blood collection. Which would you recommend for routine cord blood banking?

2. You are asked to recommend a maternity unit to start cord blood collection activities. What criteria would inform your choice of collection site?

17 HISTOCOMPATIBILITY AND IMMUNOGENETICS OF TRANSPLANTATION

The Histocompatibility and Immunogenetics (H&I) Laboratories play an important role in the selection of related and unrelated allogeneic donors for patients in need of a solid organ or haematopoietic stem cell transplantation. Their primary role in donor selection is to match donors with recipients through characterisation and matching of molecules encoded by genes of the human major histocompatibility complex, termed HLA.

17.1 The HLA System and Haematopoietic Stem Cell Transplantation

The HLA genes are located on the short arm of Chromosome 6 in a region spanning about 3500Kb. These genes have been divided into two classes according to their structure, function and cellular distribution. The HLA class I genes (HLA-A, -B and -C) code for a highly polymorphic transmembrane glycoprotein with three extracellular domains (α1, α2 and α3) which is non-covalently linked to the non-polymorphic β2-microglobulin encoded by a gene outside the HLA region on Chromosome 15. The HLA class I molecules are expressed on nearly all nucleated cells albeit at different levels and their primary function is to present short peptide fragments of about 9 amino acids from endogenous proteins to CD8 positive, cytotoxic T cells. On the other hand, the HLA class II genes (HLA-DRA, -DRB -DQA, -DQB and –DPA, -DPB) code for an heterodimer comprised of two non-covalently linked chains each with two extracellular domains and both encoded by genes within the HLA region. These class II molecules are present primarily on antigen presenting cells and their function is to present peptide fragments of variable length derived from exogenous proteins to CD4 positive helper T cells.

An important feature of the HLA genes is their extensive polymorphisms and the strong linkage disequilibrium in which alleles of these genes segregate. As a consequence of their role in acquired immune responses and the high level of polymorphism that exists within the genes, the HLA class I and II molecules provide the most important immunological barrier to tissue and haematopoietic stem cell transplantation.

17.2 Methods of HLA Typing

In order to minimise the risk of immune-mediated complications following tissues, organs and haematopoietic stem cell transplantation (i.e., graft rejection and graft versus host disease (GvHD)), the donor and recipient are matched for HLA-A, -B, -C, -DR and -DQ molecules. The classical serological technique, originally described by Terasaki and McClelland in 1964 to define these gene products has been now largely superseded by DNA techniques.

At present, the definition of the HLA class I and class II antigens also called 'tissue typing' is achieved through a variety of DNA-based techniques using the polymerase chain reaction with either sequence specific primers (PCR-SSP), sequence-specific oliginucleotides probes (PCR-SSOP) or by sequence-based typing (PCR-SBT).

One of the most commonly used techniques for class I and II typing is PCR-SSP (PCR-using sequence-specific primers). Here PCR primer pairs able to directly discriminate HLA alleles are used to directly amplify DNA of specific alleles. By using a panel of PCR primer mixtures able to amplify a range of HLA alleles a full HLA type can be determined. The method has tremendous flexibility being able to define alleles at low resolution, equivalent to serological specificity, or at high-resolution where individual alleles are discriminated.

Various other DNA-based methods have been developed but of those PCR-SSOP and sequence-based typing (PCR-SBT) are more frequently used for routine HLA typing prior to haematopoietic stem cell transplantation.

A modification of the SSOP technique where the labelled PCR products are hybridized with oliginucleotide specific probes (also called reverse SSOP or rSSOP) coupled to colour beads and the reactions read on flow cytometer based instrument the Luminex has recently been described.

Whereas serological techniques define the HLA molecules at the level of "broad" and "split" specificities of which 24 HLA-A, 50 HLA-B and 9 HLA-C have been described, the use of DNA based techniques allows the identification of these molecules at the DNA (allele) level. For example, the most common HLA-A specificity, HLA-A2, which occurs in about 50% of Caucasoid individuals, is now known to include over 200 HLA-A2 alleles. Regular updates of the number of alleles observed at each loci are found in the IMGT/HLA database (http://www.ebi.ac.uk/imgt/hla/).

17.3 HLA Nomenclature

There are two accepted nomenclature systems to allow serological specificities, such as HLA-A2 and -B44, and equivalent allele designations to be discriminated. Thus, an HLA-B allele encoding the B44 specificity might be designated HLA-B*44 (low resolution) or HLA-B*4402 (high-resolution). In this designation, HLA-B defines the locus, the asterisk separates the locus name from the allele name and digits 02 uniquely defines the B44 allele. A silent mutation that doesn't affect the amino acid sequence is designated by two further digits.

For example, HLA-A*680101 and A*680102 indicate two A*6801 alleles that differ by a single nucleotide that does not affect the amino acid sequence of the molecule. An example of the new DNA based nomenclature can be found at http://hla.alleles.org/nomenclature/naming.html.

17.4 Donor Selection in Haematopoietic Stem Cell Transplantation

As a single amino acid difference in an HLA molecule can initiate graft rejection or GvHD the choice of donor will depend, at least in part, on the level of HLA compatibility required between the donor and recipient. The first step to identify a donor is to type family members since the donor of choice would be an HLA identical sibling. In this circumstance, it is only necessary to perform low resolution HLA typing of class I (HLA-A, B and C) and class II (DRB1 and DQB1) of the patient, the siblings and both parents to determine the haplotypes. If a sibling is HLA-identical, i.e. geno-identical sharing both haplotypes, the transplant can be performed without further HLA investigations. If a sibling is a monozygotic twin, this would be a syngeneic transplant and, although this donor may be chosen, they may not be ideal in some circumstances as some of the 'graft versus leukaemia' affect may be lost leading to a high risk of disease relapse. If both parents share a common haplotype, it is possible that one of them could be identical to the patient and this would be termed a pheno-identical transplant.

However in these cases, high-resolution typing may be required to ensure HLA compatibility. Within a family if a donor has been identified with only one HLA difference, this would be termed a one antigen mismatch family donor and, although the transplant may be performed, there would be an increased risk of graft rejection or GvHD. In this circumstance it might be appropriate to deplete the graft of T cells either using Campath or CD34 of the peripheral blood stem cell (PBSC) collection. Within a family where the parents and siblings share one common haplotype with the patient, this would be termed a haploidentical transplant and the risks of rejection and GvHD would be extremely high. In this case, T cell depletion by CliniMACS™ CD34 selection would be advisable to prevent GvHD. Although mismatched related donors have an increased risk of GvHD over matched sibling donors, many centres would consider using an HLA matched unrelated donor rather than use an HLA mismatched related donor. In the past few years umbilical cord blood (UCB) has been shown to be a suitable source of HSC for transplantation. However, due to the limited doses of HSC present in the UCB collection these have been mainly used in children, although a number of protocols have now been developed including the use of two UCB collections.

To select any unrelated donor, high-resolution HLA typing of the patient is recommended as unrelated donors are more likely to possess HLA incompatibilities that are only detected using high-resolution typing such as SBT or other DNA methods With the introduction of high-resolution HLA typing for the selection of unrelated donors, it has become clear that once one allele mismatch has been identified, others are likely to occur elsewhere through linkage with other HLA genes located nearby. The number of mismatches at either low or high resolution, appear to have an additive affect in terms of GvHD and transplant related mortality.

Cord blood transplantation has been shown to be associated with less severe aGVHD and there it has been suggested that HLA matching criteria could be less stringent.

The use of HLA MM cord blood units has highlighted the relevance of donor specific antibodies in the outcome of the transplant therefore patients should be tested for the presence of these antibodies prior to the transplant using currently available techniques.

17.5 Post Transplant Monitoring

Following HSC transplants it is important to monitor engraftment of the transplanted cells. This is done by measuring the extent of donor chimerism within the recipient blood cells. A variety of micro-satellite markers encoded by genes outside the HLA region that differ in length between the donor and recipient are utilised for this purpose. In brief, discriminating micro-satellite markers are specifically amplified by the PCR and separated on polyacrymide gels. The proportion ot donor and recipient DNA can be estimated by comparing the banding patterns. This information, if gathered regularly overtime can give early warning of graft rejection or relapse allowing early intervention.

17.6 Suggested Reading

1. *Haemopoietic Stem Cell Transplantation. The EBMT Handbook.* Apperley J, Carreras E, Gluckman E, Gratwohl A, Masszi T (eds). Pages 31 to 66

2. *Essential Immunology* 9th ed. IM. Roitt. Pages 253 to 378.

3. *Practical Transfusion Medicine.* Murphy MF, Pamphilon DH (3rd Eds).

4. HLA information from Bone Marrow Donors World-wide. http://www.bmdw.org/index.php?id=hla_info

5. (http://web17110.vs.netbenefit.co.uk/HIG/data.html)

6. http://www.ebi.ac.uk/imgt/hla/

7. Takanashi M et al (2010) The impact of anti-HLA antibodies on unrelated cord blood transplantations. Blood, 116 (15); 2839-2846

17.7 Self Assessment Questions

Multiple Choice Questions

1. Which of the following statements about HPCT are true?
   a) HPCs must always be mobilised from the bone marrow space for harvesting.
   b) The therapeutic use of HPC-A products is more prevalent than HPC-M or HPC-C.
   c) HPCT is appropriate for some non-malignant conditions.
   d) HPC-A transplants are associated with more GvHD than HPC-C transplants.
   e) HPCs can be identified using cytometric assessment of CD34 expression.

2. Allogeneic adult stem cell donors are selected on the basis of:
   a) HLA match for recipient.
   b) CMV status.
   c) Physical fitness.
   d) Blood group.
   e) Ethnic background

3. Which of the following statements about GvHD are true?
   a) GvHD is mediated by CD4 and CD8 T cells.
   b) GvHD is always a chronic disorder.
   c) Matching donor and recipient at major HLA loci will prevent GvHD.
   d) GvHD and GvM are mediated by similar mechanisms.
   e) Tends to be less severe following transplantation of cord blood stem cells.

4. Which of the following statements are true of reduced intensity conditioning allogeneic transplants?
   a) They are associated with lower transplant-related mortality than regimens using high dose conditioning.
   b) They may be considered in patients with co-morbid diseases.
   c) They owe their efficacy to the use of myeloablative drugs.
   d) They are associated with a higher incidence of relapse.
   e) They may allow stem cell transplantation in older patients.

Short Answer Questions

1. What is the polymerase chain reaction and how does it work?

2. Describe the role of HLA-reactive antibodies in allogeneic stem cell transplantation?

Assignments

1. Describe the basic principles behind the HLA typing methods used in your local H&I laboratory. What are the advantages and disadvantages of these methods compared to others commonly in use?

2. What options are currently available to minimise the risks associated with HLA reactive antibodies in a recipient of an allogeneic stem cell transplant?

18 TRANSFUSION OF STEM CELL TRANSPLANT PATIENTS

18.1 Abstract

Stem cell transplant (SCT) patients frequently require intensive blood component support. Transfusions can be complicated by transmission of viral and bacterial infections, transfusion-associated GvHD, febrile non-haemolytic transfusion reactions (FNHTR) and transfusion-related acute lung injury (TRALI). Alloimmunisation (AI) to red cell antigens may cause difficulties in selecting compatible blood whilst AI to the human leucocyte antigens (HLA) present on platelets may cause refractoriness to subsequent platelet transfusions. It is essential to define robust transfusion policies and procedures; these should be regularly audited. This chapter briefly reviews the blood components available for transfusion and discusses the use of granulocyte transfusions in the setting of SCT, the impact of reduced-intensity conditioning (RIC) transplantation on transfusion requirements, the prevention of cytomegalovirus (CMV) transmission and the management of ABO-mismatched transplants.

18.2 Introduction

Recent years have seen the introduction into routine use of high quality blood components. The specification, method of preparation, storage, shelf life and mode of administration of each will be described. Indications for the use of each component in the transfusional support of patients undergoing bone marrow transplant (BMT) will be discussed.

Red cells, usually suspended in an optimal additive solution are transfused to correct anaemia due to marrow failure, haemorrhage and haemolysis aiming to keep the haemoglobin or packed cell volume (PCV) at or above predefined levels. This will ensure good tissue oxygenation. Similarly platelets are transfused to maintain the platelet count above specified thresholds.

Fresh frozen plasma (FFP) may be given to correct the abnormalities of coagulation that are observed where there is for example, liver disease resulting from GvHD or veno-occlusive disease, thrombotic thrombocytopenic purpura (TTP) or disseminated intravascular coagulation (DIC). Recently there has been increased interest in the use of both therapeutic and prophylactic granulocyte transfusions in patients with sepsis and policies for their clinical use will be described.

Transfusion may be complicated by transfusion transmitted infection (TTI) – both viral or bacterial infection, transfusion-associated GvHD, FNHTR and TRALI. In addition, alloimmunisation to red cell antigens causing difficulties in selecting compatible blood and to the human leukocyte antigens (HLA) present on platelets which may cause refractoriness to subsequent transfusions of randomly-selected platelets may occur. Amongst infectious agents transmissible by blood components, CMV is particularly important in BMT patients and strategies to minimise CMV seroconversion in susceptible recipients are defined[1].

The following sections deal systematically with:

1. Microbiological testing of donated blood;
2. Blood grouping and antibody testing;
3. CMV screening;
4. Leucodepletion of blood components;
5. Irradiation of blood components;
6. Specific pre-transplant transfusion considerations;
7. Provision of appropriate red cell, platelet, FFP and granulocyte support;
8. Policies for prevention of transfusion-induced alloimmunisation to red cells and HLA;
9. Strategies for minimising complications of transfusion.

18.3 Regulatory Framework

The European Union Directive 2002/98/EC sets standards for the collection, testing, processing, storage and distribution of human blood and blood components.[2] It requires that Blood Establishments should be licensed and this is of importance for both Blood Centres in EU countries that undertake these activities as well as hospitals that collect and issue e.g. granulocytes for transfusion. The most important aspects of the Directive are:

- The fate of each unit of all blood components should be recorded and this record kept for 30 years. i.e. vein-to-vein traceability

- Robust Quality Systems should be in place

- The processing of blood and blood components should be undertaken by licensed blood establishments (see above)

- Training should be provided for hospital transfusion laboratory staff

- Haemovigilance systems should be established to include the reporting of adverse events

Establishments are licensed by the Competent Authorities in EU Member States following inspection by a regulatory body – in the UK this is the Medicines and Healthcare Products Regulatory Authority (MHRA). Reports of compliance must be submitted.

18.4 General Policies

18.4.1 Microbiological Testing of Donated Blood

A number of microbial agents may be transmitted by blood transfusion. These include hepatitis B and C, HIV-1 and –2, HTLV-1, CMV and syphilis. In the UK Blood Services routinely carry out the following tests:

1. HbsAg, i.e. hepatitis B surface antigen*;
2. Anti-HCV*, i.e. hepatitis C antibodies;
3. HCV-Nucleic acid testing (NAT)
4. Anti-HIV 1 + 2*, i.e. HIV 1 + 2 antibodies;
5. HIV-NAT in some cases
6. Syphilis.

* mandated by the EU Directive

In addition, donations may be tested for:

1. Anti-HBc, i.e. anti-hepatitis B core antigen;
2. Alanine aminotransferase (ALT): a surrogate marker of hepatitis C;
3. Anti-HTLV-1, i.e. HTLV-1;
4. p 24 antigen for HIV-1.

There is a variation from country to country in the number of mandatory tests performed on each blood donation.

Testing for anti-CMV antibody to identify CMV seronegative donors is done on a proportion of blood donations, sufficient to identify enough CMV seronegative components for transfusion to those patients in whom it is appropriate.

Bacterial contamination is a relatively common occurrence with an incidence estimated at 0.05 – 0.5% of components[3]. The sources of bacteria are donor bacteraemia and contamination with bacteria present on the skin at the time of donation or present in blood packs. Screening tests for bacteria in platelet concentrates (PC) using automated blood culture systems e.g. BacT/ALERT have been evaluated[3] and are now used routinely by some transfusion services. PC are not issued until at least 48 hours after collection but the storage period may be extended to 7 days once sterility has been evaluated. The risk of bacterial transmission is also minimised by careful donor selection, meticulous attention to sterility during venepuncture, diversion of the first 30mL of blood collected, which contains most of the bacteria, away from the primary collection pack and sterility during preparation of blood components.   Bacterial contamination should be suspected in any patient who develops a febrile reaction characterised by fever, chills and/or hypotension.

The organisms that most frequently contaminate red cell and platelet transfusions are shown in Table 1.

Table 1. Bacteria that Most Frequently Contaminate Blood Components

Red Cells		Platelets	
Yersinia enterocolitica	51%	Staph epidermidis	25%
Pseudomonas fluorescens	27%	Staphylococcus aureus	6%
Other species	22%	Salmonella choleraesuis	14%
		Serratia marcescens	10%
		Bacillus cereus	6%
		Others	39%

Microbiological testing does not completely remove the risk of TTI; although the chance of infection in the UK after transfusion of screened blood components from known/previously tested donors is estimated to be in excess of 1 in 2×10^6 for HIV-1, HBV and HCV. This risk will vary somewhat according to the donor selection and testing policies that are operative within a Blood Service.

18.4.2 Blood Grouping and Antibody Testing

The ABO and Rhesus D type of all donated blood is determined by standard techniques. All donations are tested to exclude the presence of immune IgG antibodies that are reactive with common blood groups and which occur after an immunising stimulus such as pregnancy or transfusion. Selected units of red cells may be more extensively phenotyped (Kell, Duffy, Kidd, MNSs antigens) for patients who develop red cell alloantibodies.

18.4.3 Prevention of CMV Transmission

A proportion of SCT patients are CMV seropositive pre-transplant or have seropositive donors. They require regular screening by PCR and antigenemia testing together with ganciclovir therapy where appropriate to minimise the impact of virus reactivation and prevent clinical infection post-transplant. All CMV seronegative SCT patients with CMV seronegative donors (neg/neg) and patients with haematological and other disorders who are likely to proceed to a transplant should receive blood components that have a minimal risk of causing CMV acquisition[1]. Studies show that the use of CMV seronegative components is associated with an incidence of CMV infection in CMV neg/neg SCT of between 1-4%[4,5,6,7]. CMV is transmitted via leucocytes and leucodepletion also minimises the risk of CMV transmission[4,5,6,8]. CMV seronegative and leucodepleted blood components are probably of equivalent efficacy but this view is not generally accepted[6,9]. Further evidence from prospective randomised controlled studies (PRCT) using pre-storage leucodepleted blood components is required. Centres must establish their own policies.

18.4.4 Leucodepleted Blood Components

Transfused leucocytes cause alloimmunisation to HLA class 1 antigens in a proportion of patients. This may be manifested clinically as FNHTRs, although these may also be caused by antibodies to neutrophils, platelets, plasma proteins and by cytokines such as interleukin (IL)-1, IL-6, IL-8 and tumour necrosis factor (TNF)-alpha which accumulate in stored blood components, especially platelets. HLA alloimmunisation may cause accelerated destruction of transfused platelets that are HLA incompatible. This is clinically manifested as a failure to achieve a satisfactory increment after platelet transfusion (refractoriness). A summary of the adverse effects of transfused leucocytes is shown in Table 2.

Donor dendritic cells (DC) which are present in red cell and platelet transfusions appear to be responsible for sensitisation to HLA. Studies show that removal of leucocytes to less than 5×10^6 per transfusate prevents HLA alloimmunisation in more than 97% of patients with haematological malignancies. However, refractoriness may not be prevented since in over 50% of cases it results from increased platelet destruction due to non-immune causes which include fever, splenomegaly, DIC and amphotericin therapy etc.

HLA-alloimmunisation is also associated with a higher incidence of graft failure in patients with severe aplastic anaemia. Filtration of blood or its components is best performed in Blood Centres and hospital blood banks. Data from studies where leucocytes were filtered from blood components at the bedside show that this may be ineffective in preventing or reducing FNHTR, alloimmunisation and refractoriness.

Table 2. Adverse Effects of Transfused Leucocytes

HLA alloimmunisation causing
- FNHTR
- Refractoriness to random donor platelets
- Graft rejection
- Shortened, red cell survival
Transmission of micro-organisms
- CMV
- HTLV – 1 / 11
- Toxoplasma gondii
- Yersinia enterocolitica
Immunomodulation
- GvHD
- Activation of viruses in host cells e.g. HIV – 1
- Immune suppression of T- and NK-cell functions
Affecting the quality of stored blood
- microaggregate formation
- metabolic deterioration during storage

Indications for leucodepleted blood components include:

1. Pre-BMT in patients with SAA to reduce the likelihood of graft failure. This may also apply to patients with haemoglobinopathies but, as yet, there is insufficient evidence to be certain.
2. Pre- and post-BMT to prevent recurrent FNHTR.
3. Pre-and post-BMT to prevent HLA alloimmunisation and minimise platelet refractoriness. This is optional since there is no evidence of a significant impact on important clinical outcome measures such as survival post-BMT except in patients with SAA. Nonetheless many Blood Services have implemented leucodepletion of a large proportion or, in some cases, all of their blood components. In the UK universal leucodepletion was implemented with the aim of minimising the theoretical risk of transfusion-associated transmission of the causative agent of variant Creutzfeld-Jakob disease (vCJD).
4. As an alternative to CMV seronegative components.

18.4.5 Gamma-Irradiated Blood Components

HLA incompatible third party leucocytes contained in donated blood components can engraft and initiate an alloreactive response after transfusion. This can cause
TA-GvHD, manifest clinically by fever, rash, diarrhoea, jaundice and pancytopenia. TA-GvHD is fatal in > 90% of cases, so prevention is essential. Donor leucocytes are inactivated by gamma-irradiation of 2500 cGy and all components for BMT recipients should be irradiated from the time that conditioning therapy is started.

Further, HLA matched platelet transfusions should be irradiated as should those from family members since HLA haplotype sharing has been shown to result in TA-GVHD even in immunocompetent patients. A summary of the indications for blood component irradiation is shown in Table 3.

Table 3. Indications for Irradiated Blood Components

Indication
Allogeneic HSC recipients from time of conditioning therapy for 6 months or until the lymphocyte count is 1×10^9/L in the absence of chronic GvHD
Allogeneic HSC donors
Autologous HSC recipients (from 7 days before harvest until 3 months post transplant)
All donations from HLA-matched donors or 1st or 2nd degree relatives
All patients with Hodgkin's disease at any stage of therapy
All patients treated with purine analogues e.g. fludarabine
All patients with congenital immunodeficiency states

Higher dosages may be used with detriment to blood cell function, e.g. platelets show normal functional characteristics through 5 days storage after irradiation with 5000 cGy. Red cells leak potassium during storage and this is worsened by irradiation. Therefore, storage is limited to 14 days after 2500 cGy. TA-GvHD has been shown to occur after 1500 – 2000 cGy and this dose range is not recommended[10].

18.5 Pre-Transplant Transfusions

The following provisions apply:

1. Red cell transfusions for patients with sickle cell disease are initially matched for ABO, Rhesus D and Kell antigens but additional matching for the Rhesus CcEe and for Duffy (Fya,Fyb), Kell (Kk), Kidd (Jka, Jkb) and MNSs antigens may be required if alloantibodies have formed.

2. Leucodepleted blood components should be transfused to all patients with aplastic anaemia.

3. Either CMV seronegative or leucodepleted blood components should be transfused to susceptible patients to prevent CMV acquisition.

4. Blood components should be gamma-irradiated for peripheral blood progenitor cell transplant patients during stem cell mobilisation and collection since transfused leucocytes might be captured in the PBPC harvest and subsequently induce TA-GvHD.

5. Blood components transfused to allogeneic marrow donors immediately pre- or intra-operatively should also be irradiated.

18.6 Red Cell Transfusions

The following definitions for red cells, platelet concentrates, FFP, cryoprecipitate and granulocyte products are derived from the Guidelines for UK Blood Services.

Red cells may be:

1. Suspended in OAS, usually a combination of saline, adenine, glucose and mannitol (SAG-M): PCV 50 – 70%; volume 220 – 420 ml. This is the product of choice.
2. Derived from whole blood from which a proportion of the plasma has been removed – plasma reduced blood (PRB): PCV 50 – 60%; volume 200 – 450 ml.
3. Unmodified whole blood: volume 420 – 520 ml. This last term is misleading since platelets and labile coagulation factors deteriorate rapidly in stored blood.

The storage period is 35 – 42 days at 4 ± 2°C.

18.6.1 Transfusion Policy

1. Red cells should be matched for ABO and Rhesus D type.
2. Extended phenotyping may be necessary in some patients, e.g. those with sickle cell disease.
3. Red cells should be cross-matched against the patient's serum by standard techniques prior to transfusion.
4. Thresholds should be defined for haemoglobin and PCV below which red cell transfusions are always given. Suggested arbitrary cut off points are Hb less than 8.0 g/dL and PCV less than 25%.
5. In adults 1 unit of red cells raises the Hb by 1.0 g/dL whereas in children the volume of blood to be transfused is derived from the formula:

    Volume = Increase in Hb (g/dL) required x 4 x weight (kg)

These policies apply both to SCT patients as well as being accepted recommendations for patients with bone marrow failure who require supportive transfusions.

18.7 Platelet Transfusions

Platelet concentrates (PCs) can be made in three ways:

1. By centrifuging units of whole blood in a 'top- top' pack format to obtain platelet rich plasma (PRP), which is then further concentrated. PRP-PCs may be transfused individually or pooled in multiples - usually 6. The mean platelet content per pool is 3.4×10^{11} and the mean contamination with white blood cells is 365×10^{6}.
2. By centrifuging units of whole blood in a 'bottom & top' pack format to separate the buffy coat (BC), pooling 4 BCs and recentrifuging to separate PRP which is then expressed into a secondary storage container. The mean platelet content per pool is 3.2×10^{11} and the mean contamination with white blood cells is 5.7×10^{6}.
3. By collecting PCs directly on a cell separator. Dual arm, continuous flow apheresis is preferred and some cell separators collect PCs with an inherently low WBC content. The mean platelet content per pool is 3.15×10^{11} and the mean contamination with white blood cells is 0.3×10^{6}.

    The storage period is 5 days at 22 ± 2°C.
    (All data generated by the NHSBT, Bristol Centre, UK).

These policies apply both to SCT patients as well as being accepted recommendations for patients with bone marrow failure who require supportive transfusions.

18.7.1 Transfusion Policy

1. PCs should be ABO and Rh compatible wherever possible.

2. ABO incompatibility may reduce the expected count increment (CI) by 10 – 30%.

3. Group O PCs should be tested for high titre anti-A, B and if positive should only be transfused to group O recipients to avoid haemolysis caused by passive administration of antibody.

4. If Rh D positive platelets are given to an Rh D negative patient it is reasonable to give 250 iu polyclonal anti-Rh (D) immunoglobulin. Since the chance of Rh immunisation is probably less than 5% this may be omitted and the patients serum screened for immune red cell antibodies, or prior to a red cell transfusion.

5. Studies show that a threshold of 10×10^9/L in stable thrombocytopenic patients is optimal for prophylactic platelet transfusion. Until recently most BMT patients were transfused PCs when the platelet count was less than 20×10^9/L.

6. A higher threshold of 20×10^9/L should be used in patients with fever, sepsis, splenomegaly and other well established causes of increased platelet consumption.

7. If an invasive procedure is planned, e.g. central line insertion, the platelet count should be $> 50 \times 10^9$/L.

8. PCs should be transfused when there is significant clinical bleeding, irrespective of the platelet count. PCs are contraindicated in patients with TTP.

9. In adults the usual dose of platelets is 3×10^{11} (adult therapeutic dose – ATD) in a volume of 200 – 300 ml.

10. Children > 30 kg receive one ATD. Children < 30 kg are given 10ml kg.

11. Rate of transfusion:

    - adults 1 ATD is given in less than 60 minutes.

    - children e.g. 2 – 5 ml/kg/hr.

The outcome of platelet transfusions can be monitored by:

1. Looking for cessation of bleeding.

2. Measuring the platelet count the following day. A persistent value $< 20 \times 10^9$L suggests refractoriness.

3. Measuring the platelet count at between 10 – 60 minutes post-transfusion – the CI. A corrected (C) CI is calculated as follows:

$$CCI = \frac{CI \times 10^9/L \times surface\ area\ (m2)}{Platelets\ transfused \times 10^{11}}$$

The CCI should be more than 7.5.

If the patient is refractory to transfusion of PCs, samples should be taken to test for HLA antibodies. If these are detected, HLA-matched platelets collected by apheresis of HLA-typed donors should be used in these patients.

If the CCI is less than 7.5 following transfusion of HLA matched PCs and the patient is not bleeding then withhold platelet transfusions.

If the CCI using well-HLA-matched PCs is less than 7.5 and/or bleeding persists then:

1. Check for non-immune causes of refractoriness. If refractoriness is due to non-immune causes, particularly if there is significant clinical bleeding then either give 2 or 3 ATD or give 1 ATD twice or three times daily.

2. Look for platelet-specific antibodies – this is a rare cause of refractoriness in BMT patients.

3. Consider using cross-matched platelets. HLA-typed or random units or platelets are cross-matched against the patient's serum usually by an immunofluorescent technique and non-reactive units selected if possible[11].

18.8 FFP And Cryoprecipitate Transfusion

FFP is made by centrifuging whole blood and freezing separated plasma within 6 hours of collection. The volume is 200 - 340 ml and the Factor VIII level should be greater than 70 iu/ml.

Cryoprecipitate is made by thawing FFP at 4°C and collecting the precipitate that forms by further centrifugation in a volume of approximately 20 - 30 ml. This is then refrozen. The fibrinogen content should be greater than 140 mg/dL and the Factor VIII level greater than 70 iu/ml. FFP and cryoprecipitate have a storage period of 12 months at -30°C.

18.8.1 Transfusion Policy

FFP transfusion (at a volume of 10-15 ml/kg) is indicated after BMT:

1. As replacement fluid in TTP where plasma exchange is undertaken.
2. In the presence of liver disease causing significant defects of coagulation factors.
3. In severe DIC.

FFP transfusion may also be indicated after BMT where a large volume blood transfusion, e.g. after haemorrhage, has caused a dilutional coagulopathy.

Cryoprecipitate transfusion is indicated in severe DIC when the fibrinogen is <100 mg/dL.

The outcome of FFP and cryoprecipitate transfusion should be monitored by measuring the prothombin time (PT) and activated partial thromboplastin time (APTT). The ratios compared to control should correct to less than 1.5. In DIC the fibrinogen should be greater than 100 mg/dL.

18.9 Granulocyte Transfusions

Granulocytes are collected by apheresis of healthy donors who may be family members or unrelated volunteers. The granulocyte content is greater than 10×10^9/unit but the volume may be variable. Granulocyte products must be irradiated prior to transfusion.

18.9.1 Transfusion Policy

Granulocyte transfusions (GT) are prepared by pooling buffy coats from whole blood donations or they may be collected by the apheresis of steady state healthy donors who may be family members or unrelated volunteers. Granulocyte apheresis donors must have a full medical assessment and testing to select those that are ABO compatible and CMV appropriate. The granulocyte content is in the range 5-10 x 10^9/unit for both these preparations. Mobilised granulocytes can be collected from donors who receive G-CSF (5-10 micrograms/Kg) and/or dexamethasone (8mg) – both given 12-24 hours before - to increase the number that can be collected during a standard apheresis procedure. Current practice is to give only G-CSF since the use of steroids has been associated with the development of posterior subcapsular cataracts[12] and the two methods give similar yields[13].This strategy gives a granulocyte yield of 10-100 x 10^9 per unit and data available so far indicates that significant granulocyte increments e.g. 1-2 x10^9/l can be obtained[14]. By contrast it is unusual to observe such increments with buffy coat or unmobilised granulocytes. All granulocyte products must be irradiated prior to transfusion to prevent TA-GvHD. Cross-matching is also required. A recent Cochrane Systemic Review indicated that there is currently inconclusive evidence from PRCTs to support or refute the use of GT in neutropenic patients. Further PRCT are required before definitive recommendations can be made[15]. There is recent anecdotal evidence that prophylactic administration of granulocytes may reduce the incidence of severe fungal infections after BMT but currently few centres use such transfusions and further studies are needed[14]. Furthermore, granulocyte transfusions increase the likelihood of HLA immunisation and platelet refractoriness. Granulocyte transfusions are probably best reserved for patients with granulocyte counts less than 0.2 x 10^9/L and documented bacterial or fungal infections not responding to at least 3 days of appropriate antimicrobial therapy, in situations where the granulocyte count is not expected to recover within 7 days.

18.10 Donor/Recipient ABO Incompatibility and Transfusion Support

Approximately 15 – 25% of HLA identical sibling donor/recipient pairs differ for ABO blood groups and the figure is higher in alternative donor transplants. In myeloablative transplants ABO incompatibility is associated with an increase risk of delayed red cell engraftment, pure red cell aplasia (PRCA), haemolysis and increased transfusion requirements[16]. There are also reports of increased platelet transfusion requirements. ABO mismatch does not affect neutrophil engraftment, the incidence of graft rejection, GvHD, disease progression or overall survival[17].

RIC transplants are associated with decreased RCC and PC usage[16] and it has been demonstrated with chimerism studies that early erythroid progenitors engrafted as promptly as myeloid progenitors[18] However, as with myeloablative SCT, engraftment of mature red cells is delayed, cases of PRCA have also been reported and ABO mismatch is associated with increased red cell transfusion requirements[19]. Recipient plasma cells produce anti – donor ABO alloagglutinins and after RIC SCT the rate of decline of anti-donor haemagglutinins takes twice as long and this can lead to more haemolysis[20]. In one report of 40 patients who had RIC SCT, ABO mismatch was associated with one death due to haemolysis, 3 cases of PRCA, 6 cases of thrombotic microangiopathy (3 fatal), an increase in rehospitalisation days, relapse or disease progression and higher TRM[21]. By contrast other reports do not show an inferior outcome[18-20].

Definitions

- Major ABO incompatibility is defined as the presence in the recipients plasma of anti- A, -B or –A,B alloagglutinins reactive with the donor's red cells, e.g. donor group A and recipient group O.

- Minor ABO incompatibility is defined as the presence of anti-A,-B or –A,B alloagglutinins in the donors plasma reactive with the recipient's red cells, e.g. donor group O and recipient group A.

- Major plus minor, also referred to as bidirectional, ABO compatibility is defined as the presence in both the donor and recipients plasma of anti-A, -B or –A,B alloagglutinins reactive with recipient and donor cells respectively, e.g. donor group A and recipient group B.

18.10.1   Incompatible stem cell graft infusion

If the titre of anti-A and/or anti-B), is less than 1:64 then bone marrow or PBPC grafts may be infused without any modification At higher titres red cells should be removed from the graft. Marrow processing or PBPC collection on certain apheresis machines such as the GAMBRO Spectra, usually results in red cell contamination of less than 5ml and ABO incompatibility may be ignored Likewise, stem cells that are separated on density gradients and washed can also be infused without regard to ABO incompatibility.

Plasma may be removed from the transplant in cases of minor ABO mismatch where the alloagglutinin titre is high to avoid acute haemolysis in the recipient. Delayed haemolytic transfusion reactions may follow the infusion of donor HSC where there is a minor ABO mismatch. This is because of a secondary (anamnestic) immune response mediated via memory B cells in the graft against recipient ABO antigens. A rise in anti-A, -B or –A,B titre is seen together with anaemia and jaundice. This phenomenon is rarely, if ever, seen when bone marrows are depleted of alloreactive T-lymphocytes using strategies such as alemtuzumab (CAMPATH-1) antibody or CD34 positive cell selection since B-cells are also depleted.

18.10.2   Blood groups used for transfusion support

Before transplant recipient-type red cells and platelets should be given but after the transplant the situation is more complicated (see Figure 1)
- For major ABO mismatch use group O red cells products, irrespective of ABO group until recipient ABO antibodies are undetectable and the antiglobulin test is negative and platelets and plasma from donors of the recipients ABO type until recipient red cells no longer detected.

- For minor ABO mismatch use red cells of the donor type i.e. group O throughout. Give platelets and plasma of recipient type until recipient-type red cells are no longer detected.

- For major and minor ABO mismatch use group O red cells until recipient ABO antibodies are undetectable and the antiglobulin test is negative and then switch to donor type. For platelets and plasma use group AB until recipient red cells are undetectable.

Following graft rejection, revert to recipient-type red cells and platelets.

                    150

Fig. 1 Strategy for the Provision of Blood Components for ABO Mismatched SCT Patients

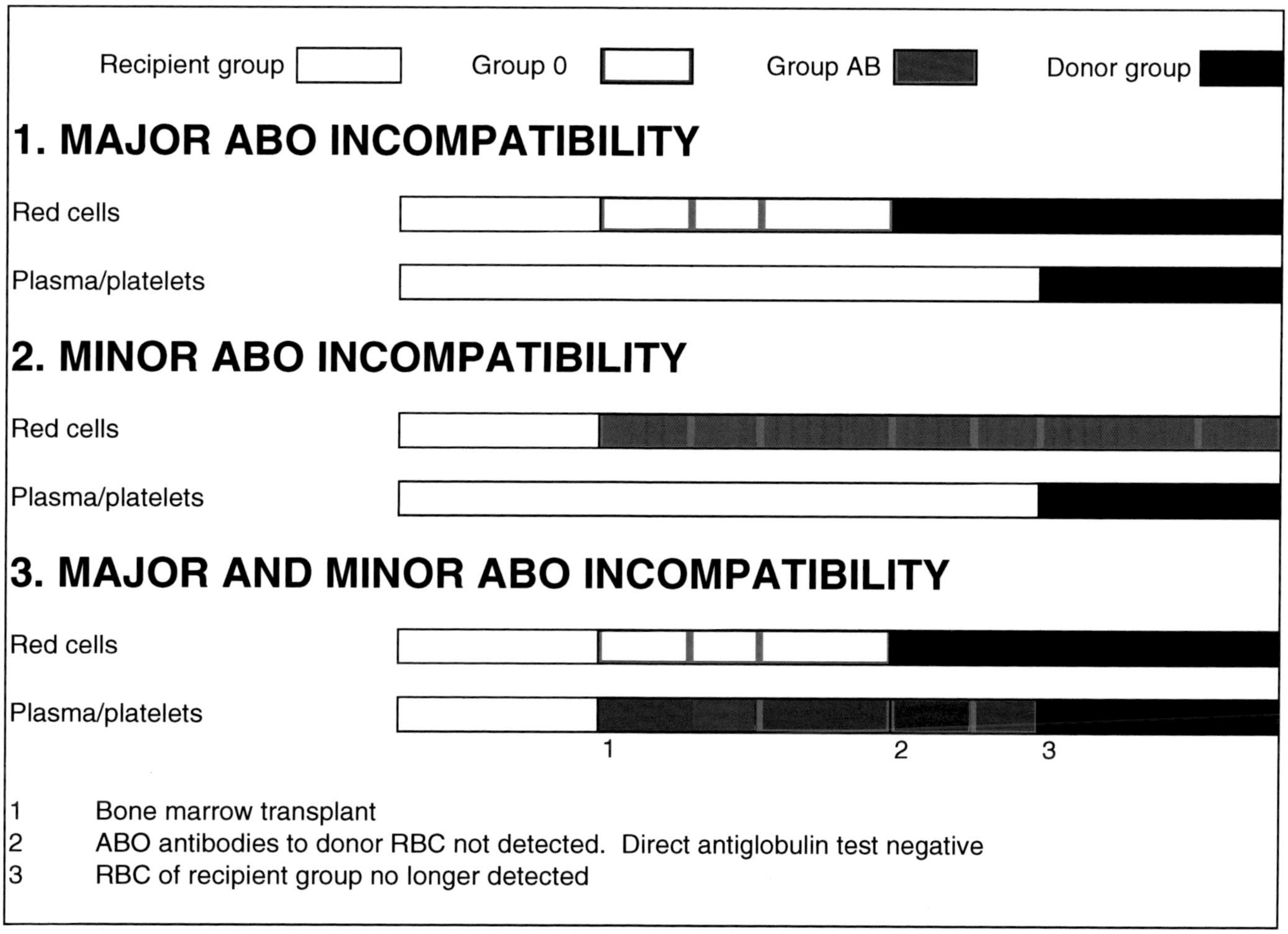

18.11 Conclusion

Transfusion support in BMT patients requires special consideration and carefully defined policies. The use of high quality blood components which have a high degree of microbiological safety and which are also gamma-irradiated and, in addition, may be CMV seronegative and leucodepleted provides optimum transfusion support and minimises the chance of adverse effects.

Acknowledgements
This chapter is based on the chapter on transfusion support first published in The EBMT Handbook 2008 with permission of the EBMT[22] and in the Education Programme of the 14th Congress of the European Hematology Association (2009).

18.12 References and Suggested Reading

18.12.1   References

1. Pamphilon DH. et al. Prevention of transfusion-transmitted cytomegalovirus infection. Transfusion Medicine. 9:115-123 (1999).

2. European Union Directive 2002/98/EC - http://eurlex.europa.eu/LexUriServ/site/en/oj/2003/l_033/l_03320030208en003000 40.pdf

3. Ramirez-Arcos S, Jenkins C, Dion J et al. Canadian experience with detection of bacterial contamination in apheresis platelets. Transfusion 2007 Mar; 47(3): 421-9

4. Bowden RA, Slichter SJ; Sayers M, et al. A comparison of filtered leukocyte-reduced and cytomegalovirus (CMV) seronegative blood products for the prevention of transfusion – associated CMV infection after marrow transplant. Blood.1995; 86: 3598-603

5. Ljungman P, Larsson K, Kumlien G, et al. Leukocyte depleted, unscreened blood products give a low risk for CMV infection and disease in CMV seronegative allogeneic stem cell transplant recipients with seronegative stem cell donors. Scand J Infect Dis 2002;34:347-50.

6. Nichols WG, Price TH, Gooley T et al. Transfusion-transmitted cytomegalovirus infection after receipt of leukoreduced blood products. Blood 2003 May 15; 101(10): 4195-200

7. Foot, Pamphilon D, Caul EO et al. Cytomegalovirus infection in recipients of related and unrelated donor bone marrow transplants no evidence of increased incidence in patients receiving unrelated donor grafts. British journal of haematology . 1998; 102:671 – 7.

8. Ronghe MD. Foot AB, Cornish JM, et al. The impact of Transfusion of leukodepleted platelet concentrates on CMV disease after allogeneic stem cell transplantation. British journal of Haematology. 2002; 118: 1124-7.

9. Narvios AB, de Lima M, Shah H et al. Transfusion of leukoreduced cellular blood components from cytomegalovirus-unscreened donors in allogeneic hematopoietic transplant recipients: analysis of 72 recipients. Bone Marrow Transplantation 2005 Sep; 36(6): 499-501

10. BCSH Blood Transfusion Task Force. Guidelines on gamma irradiation of blood components for the prevention of transfusion-associated graft-versus-host disease. Transfusion Medicine 6:261-271 (1996).

11. Murphy MF. Transfusion management of patients alloimmunized to platelet and leukocyte antigens. In, *Modern Transfusion Medicine*. Ed. D H Pamphilon. CRC Press Inc. (1995)

12. Brocklebank JT, Harcourt RB, Meadow SR. Corticosteroid – induced cataracts in idiopathic nephrotic syndrome. Arch Dis Child.1982;57:30-4

13. Heufth HG, Goudeva L, Sel S, Blasczyk R. Equivalent mobilization and collection of granulocytes for transfusion after administration of glycosylated G-CSF (3 µg/kg) plus dexamethasone versus glycosylated G-CSF (12 µg/kg) alone. Transfusion.2002;42:928-34.

14. Kerr JP, Liakopoulou E, Brown J, et al. The use of stimulated granulocyte transfusions to prevent recurrence of past severe infections after allogeneic stem cell transplantation. British Journal of Haematology 2003; Oct; 123(1); 114-8

15. Stanworth SJ, Massey E, Hyde C et al. Granulocyte transfusions for treating infections in patients with neutropenia or neutrophil dysfunction. Cochrane Database Syst. Rev. 2005 Jul 20; (3): CD005339

16. Weissinger F, Sandmaier BM, Maloney DG et al. Decreased transfusion requirements for patients receiving nonmyeloablative compared with conventional peripheral blood stem cell transplants from HLA-identical siblings. Blood 2001 Dec 15; 98 (13): 3584-8

17. Helbig G, Stella-Holowiecka B, Wojnar J et al. Pure red-cell aplasia following major and bi-directional ABO-incompatible allogeneic stem cell transplantation: recovery of donor-derived erythropoiesis after long-term treatment using different therapeutic strategies. Ann Hematol 2007 May 8; (Epub ahead of print)

18. Maciej Zaucha J, Mielcarek M, Takatu A et al. Engraftment of early erythroid progenitors is not delayed after non-myeloablative major ABO-incompatible haematopoietic stem cell transplantation. British Journal of Haematology 2002 Dec; 119(3): 740-50

19. Canals C, Muniz-Diaz E, Martinez C et al. Impact of ABO incompatibility on allogeneic peripheral blood progenitor cell transplantation after reduced intensity conditioning. Transfusion 2004 Nov; 44(11): 1603-11

20. Griffith LM, McCoy JP, Bolan CD et al. Persistence of recipient plasma cells and anti-donor isohaemagglutinins in patients with delayed donor erythropoiesis after major ABO incompatible non-myeloablative haematopoietic cell transplantation. British Journal of Haematology 2005 Mar; 128(5): 668-75

21. Worel N, Kalhs P, Keil F et al. ABO mismatch increases transplant-related morbidity and mortality in patients given nonmyeloablative allogeneic HPC transplantation. Transfusion 2003 Aug; 43(8): 1153-61

22. Pamphilon DH. Transfusion Policy in the EBMT Handbook. 5th Edition. Haemopoietic Stem Cell Transplantation. 2008.pp146-162

18.12.2 Suggested Reading

1. Anderson NA. et al. A prospective randomised study of three types of platelet concentrates in patients with haematological malignancy: corrected platelet count increments and frequency of nonhaemolytic febrile transfusion reactions. Transfusion Medicine 7:33-39 (1996).

2. Blajchman MA. Immunomodulation and blood transfusion. Am J Ther 2002 Sep-Oct; 9(5): 389-95

3. Blajchman MA The clinical benefits of the leukoreduction of blood products.. J Trauma. 2006 Jun; 60(6Suppl): S83-90.

4. Slichter SJ. Platelet refractoriness and alloimmunization. Leukemia.1998 Sep; 12 Suppl 1:S51-3

5. Williamson LM, Wimperis JZ, Williamson P et al. Bedside filtration of blood products in the prevention of HLA alloimmunization- a prospective randomised study. Alloimmunisation Study Group. Blood.1994; 83:3028 – 35

6. BCSH. Blood Transfusion Task Force Guidelines on the clinical use of leucocyte-depleted blood components. Transf Med 1998;8: 59-71. 3.

7. Stanworth SJ, Hyde C, Heddle N et al. Prophylactic platelet transfusion for haemorrhage after chemotherapy and stem cell transplantation. Cochrane Database Syst. Rev. 2004 Oct 18; (4): CD004269

8. Wandt H, Schaefer-Eckart K, Frank M et al. A therapeutic platelet transfusion strategy is safe and feasible in patients after autologous peripheral blood stem cell transplantation. Bone Marrow Transplantation 2006 Feb; 37(4): 387-92.

18.13 Self Assessment Questions

Multiple Choice Questions

1. Which of the following may occur as a result of HLA alloimmunisation?
   a) Refractoriness to random donor platelets
   b) Graft Rejection
   c) Graft versus host disease
   d) Febrile non-haemolytic transfusion reactions
   e) Reactivation of CMV infection

2. Fresh frozen plasma may be indicated post SCT in which of the following circumstances?
   a) As a replacement fluid following plasma exchange for TTP
   b) Following any autologous stem cell transplant
   c) Following the infusion of donor lymphocytes
   d) In severe disseminated intravascular coagulation
   e) To treat coagulopathy secondary to large volume blood transfusion

3. Granulocyte transfusions may be indicated in which of the following circumstances?
   a) For all neutropenic patients following SCT
   b) For all patients with bacterial infections following SCT
   c) For neutropenic patients with severe fungal infections not responding to antimicrobial therapy
   d) For patients receiving G-CSF
   e) For patients with pulmonary shadowing on chest X ray prior to SCT

4. It is recommended to remove ABO incompatible red cells from a BM graft in which of the following circumstances?
   a) The recipient has IgG anti-A or IgG anti-B antibodies
   b) The donor has IgG anti-A or IgG anti-B antibodies
   c) The recipient has anti-A or anti-B antibodies with a titre of greater than 4
   d) The recipient has anti-A or anti-B antibodies with a titre of greater than 64
   e) Any HPC, Apheresis collection containing more than 5mL ABO incompatible red cells

Short Answer Questions

1. What thresholds are used to guide the use of platelets in BMT patients?

2. What is the mechanism of immune-mediated haemolysis post ABO-incompatible BMT?

Assignments

1. By researching the available literature, determine what thresholds are used to guide the use of platelets in BMT patients? How should patients be monitored to ensure that this therapy is effective?

2. Describe the mechanisms of immune mediated haemolysis post ABO-incompatible BMT. Describe possible graft manipulations which may be used to prevent it.

TISSUE TRANSPLANTATION SCIENCE

19 COLLECTION AND RETRIEVAL OF TISSUE

Tissues can be obtained from two separate donation sources:

Living donors – removal of tissues such as bone allograft through planned primary hip operations and amniotic membrane (placental tissue) from elective caesareans;

Deceased donors – donation after death of a wide range of tissues such as corneas, bone and heart tissue for heart valves.

19.1 Living Donors

19.1.1 Introduction

Donations from living donors are collected in accordance with the requirements of relevant legislation, i.e. The Human Tissue Act 2004, and The Human Tissue Act 2006 (Scotland); and the Data Protection Act 1998.

19.1.2 Consent

Appropriate consent is the fundamental principle of the Human Tissue Acts. Consent from a living donor is obtained during a one to one discussion with the donor and a specifically trained and competent Health Care Professional. Consent is obtained from all living donors during this discussion. The consent covers all aspects of the process from agreeing for the donation of the tissue and subsequent storage, to obtain and test a blood sample for mandatory microbiological markers and also the process that will be followed in the event of a positive result. The donor also agrees that their GP may be contacted if necessary to obtain further detail if required. During the consent process a full medical and behavioural lifestyle is completed to ensure any contraindications can be identified that may affect the quality and safety of the tissue donated. It is important that consent is not taken when the patient is under the influence of certain drugs e.g. morphine for pain relief, nor undertaken by an individual who may be able to be seen to coerce the patient into donating.

19.1.3 Surgical Bone (Femoral Head) Donations

During routine hip replacement surgery the femoral head bone is removed so that a new prosthetic joint can be fitted. This bone can be donated to benefit other patients. The donation does not affect any aspect of the surgery, as the bone has to be removed anyway.

Prior to hip replacement surgery, potential donors are approached to ascertain whether they would be willing to donate their femoral head. A trained nurse or health care professional will discuss the donation process and complete the one to one consent and medical and behavioural history documentation.

The femoral head will be removed aseptically during the surgical procedure. Bone chips will be taken for bacteriological testing prior to storing the femoral head in a pre-sterile pot. All steps within the donation procedure are documented to ensure there is a full audit trail for times, consumables and individuals involved in the donation process.

Femoral heads must be frozen to –20°C or lower for up to 6 months and then to – 40°C or lower until the tissue reaches the expiry date.

19.1.4 Amniotic Membrane (Placental Tissue) Donations

Amniotic membrane is the thin membrane that covers the placenta and baby before it is born. It has many properties that make it ideal for use as a transplant material, especially for diseases or injuries affecting the ocular surface. Amniotic membrane is retrieved following the safe delivery of a baby by elective caesarean section.

Prior to elective caesareans, potential donors are approached to ascertain whether they would be willing to donate their placenta. A trained health care professional will discuss the donation process and complete the one to one consent and medical and behavioural history documentation.

The placenta will be kept as sterile as possible during the procedure and is stored in a pre-sterile pot. All steps within the donation procedure are documented to ensure there is a full audit trail for times, consumables and individuals involved in the donation process.

Placentas for subsequent processing into amniotic membrane grafts must be processed with 24 hours of donation. The donation must be placed at a temperature of 0 – 10°C within 4 hours of retrieval.

19.1.5 Heart Valve Donations

Patients undergoing a heart transplantation are able to donate their heart for valve donation. Prior to surgery, potential donors are approached to ascertain whether they would be willing to donate their heart. A trained health care professional will discuss the donation process and complete the one to one consent and medical and behavioural history documentation. The heart tissue is removed aseptically during the transplant surgery and placed in sterile packaging. All steps within the donation procedure are documented to ensure there is a full audit trail for times, consumables and individuals involved in the donation process.

Heart valve donations for subsequent processing must be processed with 24 hours of donation. The donation must be placed at a temperature of 0 – 10°C within 4 hours of retrieval.

19.1.6 Umbilical Cord Blood Donations

See chapter 16.

19.1.7 Who Can Donate Tissues?

Almost anybody can be considered for tissue donation. Unlike deceased tissue donation, there are no age restrictions.

There are however, a number of medical and behavioural contraindications, which are highlighted and discussed during the consent process. Table 1 details the main contraindications to donation with a full list available in the Tissue Donor Selection Guidelines (www.transfusionguidelines.org.uk/livedonorsoftissue).

Table 1 – Basic Contraindications to Live Tissue Donation

1. Cancer 2. Blood Transfusion (since 1980) 3. Parkinson's Disease 4. Neurological Diseases	5. Positive Mandatory Microbiological Marker 6. Positive Lifestyle risk e.g. i.v. drug user	7. Autoimmune disease 8. Tissue / Organ recipient 9. Prion associated diseases

19.2 Deceased Donors

19.2.1 Consent

Appropriate consent is the fundamental principle of the Human Tissue Acts. Communicating with the acutely bereaved about the process of donation after death is a complex area of clinical practice and as such must only be undertaken by specially trained health care professionals such as a tissue donor co-ordinator or donor transplant co-ordinator.

Consent that has been given by the deceased whilst alive and competent (e.g. carrying a organ donor card) or following their death by a nominated representative or a family member with the highest-ranking available qualifying relationship (as defined by the Human Tissue Authority) must be fully documented in writing and/or digital voice recording (were applicable). This consent will be stored as evidence. A health care professional, specially trained and directly employed to facilitate donation after death must explain the request for donation in individualised understandable terms that meets the needs of the family. They must also be satisfied that the family has been given the information they need and/or want in order to reach an informed decision about the donation. It is the responsibility of the health care professional to ensure that the family has an opportunity to express concerns and ask questions.

Depending on the circumstances of the deceased donor's death, consent may also have to be sought from the Coroner (Procurator Fiscal in Scotland) or designated deputy. This needs to be fully documented and stored as evidence as consent within the individual donation file.

19.2.2 Contra-indications to donation

Almost everybody can be considered for tissue donation, however there are age restrictions on individual tissues:

- Bone (structural)   17 -50 years
- Bone (non-structural)   no defined age limits
- Skin   no defined age limits
- Meniscus/Osteochondral   17 – 50 years
- Tendons   17 – 60 years
- Heart Valves (aortic valves)   32 week gestation – 60 years
- Heart Valves (pulmonary valves) 32 week gestation – 65 years
- Costal Cartilage   10-40 years
- Eyes (cornea donation)   if donor < 3 years, contact Eye Bank

(information source www.transfusionguidelines.org.uk, however individual tissue establishments may reduce the age limits set)

There are also a number of medical and behavioural contraindications, which are highlighted and discussed with the nominated representative(s) during the consent procedure. Examples include degenerative neurological diseases, multi-system active auto-immune diseases, infectious disease risk factors (same as blood donors) and CJD risk factors (classical and variant).

Guidelines for tissue acceptability are kept under constant review and it is essential that the most up to date guidelines are used by the Health Care Professional.

19.2.3 Basic Anatomy

Anatomy (from the Greek word Anatome meaning dissection) is the study of the structure of the body and the relationship of its constituent parts to each other. A subject, such as anatomy, with its focus on description necessarily requires a very large number of names for structures and processes. For ease, anatomists have defined 'the anatomical position' as a reference for describing parts of the body in relation to others. The anatomical position is described as the body being upright, facing forwards, with the palms of the hand also facing forwards (see diagram 1)

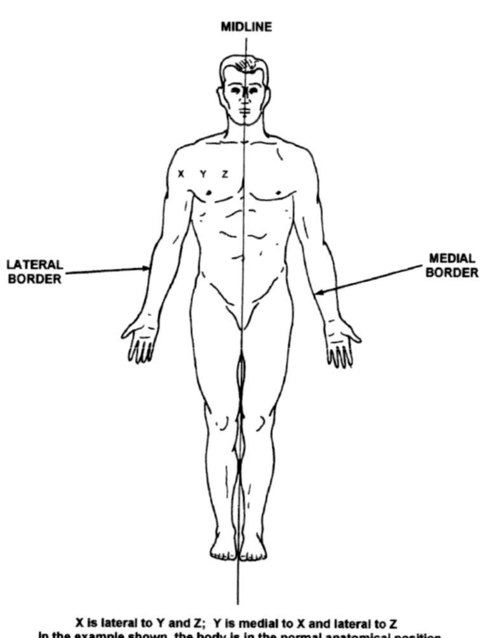

Diagram 1 – The Anatomical Position

Standardised terms of reference are used by anatomists to describe the location of a body part in relation to another. When using directional terms, it is always assumed that the body is in the anatomical position (see table 2).

Table 2 – Relative Directional Terms

Superior (The hip is *superior* to the knee)	Inferior (The ankle is *inferior* to the knee)
Anterior (The toes are *anterior* to the heel)	Posterior (The heel is *posterior* to the toes)
Medial (The nose is *medial* to the eyes)	Lateral (The eyes are *lateral* to the nose)
Proximal (The shoulder is *proximal* to the wrist)	Distal (The toes are *distal* to the hip)
Superficial (The patella ligament is *superficial* to the knee joint)	Deep (The knee joint is *deep* to the patella ligament)

19.2.4 Musculoskeletal tissue

For iliac crest donation, a 6 inch incision is made along each side of the pelvis. The bone is removed and tight suture line is made over the incisions.

For femoral head, femur and knee donation, an incision is made along the side of both legs. The bones are removed and replaced by prosthesis and padding. Tight suture lines are made over the incisions to ensure that the reconstruction leaves the body in as close to original condition as possible (Figure 1).

Figure 1 Bone donation

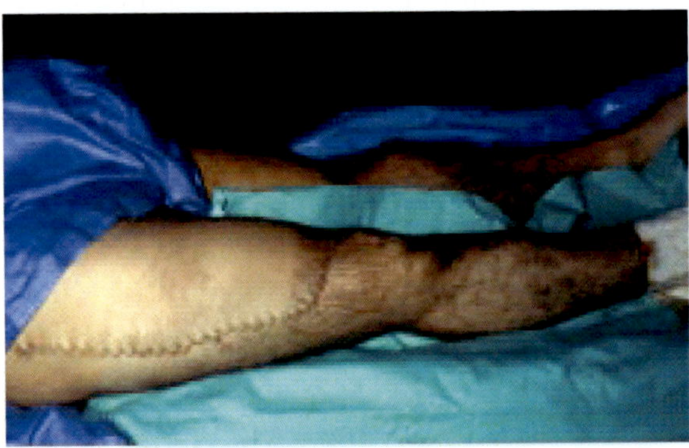

Although all musculoskeletal tissue is located as part of the endoskeleton underneath the skin, incisions into the skin can lead to possible contamination of the bone and tendons. Consequently, skin is decontaminated prior to any incision being made. Musculoskeletal tissues retrieved include the femoral head, the femoral shaft, the entire knee joint (distal femur, proximal tibia, meniscus and patella tendon), the Achilles tendon and the semi-tendinosus tendon. All bone tissue retrieved from deceased donors is processed and sterilised (normally with irradiation), either freeze dried or frozen. Femoral heads, whose cartilage has been damaged through ageing or wear and tear, but whose underlying bone is still of good quality, are also retrieved from living donors and simply stored frozen. Meniscus is retrieved, processed and stored in a cryopreserved state.

Contraindications for musculoskeletal donations are summarised in Table 3.

Table 3. Contraindications for Musculoskeletal Donation

Factor	Indicator
Time limits	Retrieved up to 48 hours post asystole
Specific	Presence of: • History of, or current malignancy (except treated Carcinoma in situ of the cervix and basal cell carcinoma of the skin); • Sepsis; • Active Multi system auto-immune diseases; • Excessive trauma to skin e.g. glass, lacerations. • Excessive trauma to bones e.g. fractures, sharp bones • Metal in-situ from previous surgery

19.2.5 Skin tissue

Skin is donated from the back of the body, from the shoulders to the ankles and from the front of the legs. Skin is removed using a dermatome (Figure 3). Donated skin for burns treatment is not full thickness (Figure 2) and there is a risk of some fluid leakage following donation (see below).

Figure 2. Donated Skin **Figure 3. Battery operated Dermatome**

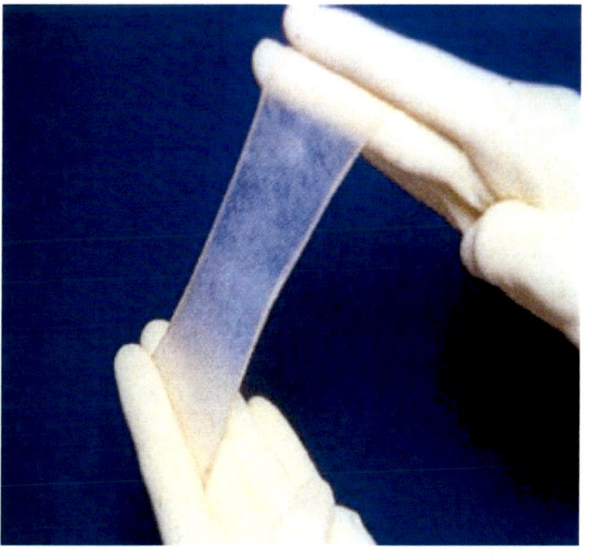

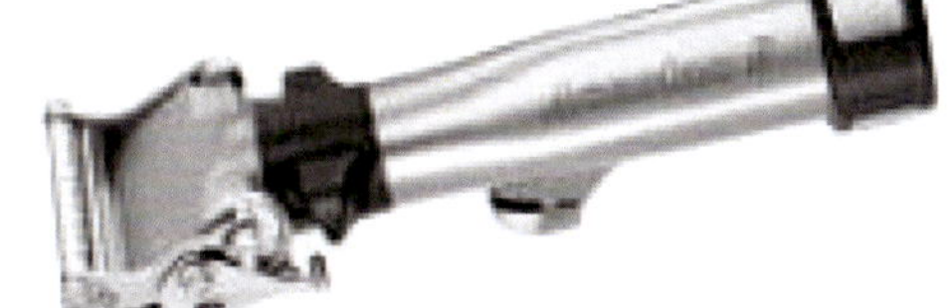

Contraindications for skin donations are summarised in Table 4.

Table 4. Contraindications for Skin Donation

Factor	Indicator
Time limits	Retrieved up to 48 hours post asystole
Specific	Presence of: • History of, or current malignancy (except treated Carcinoma in situ of the cervix and basal cell carcinoma of the skin); • Sepsis; • Active Multi system auto-immune diseases; • Severe skin disease, seek advice if unsure • Excessive or abnormally looking moles; • Excessive trauma to skin e.g. glass, lacerations. • Death caused by drowning

19.2.6 Cardiac tissue

Once the heart has been retrieved, the heart must be inverted to allow the blood contained within the heart to drain out. The heart can then be wrapped in chlorohexidine soaked gauze. One member of the team should then open a drape and hold it over the sterile field, while the other team member places the heart inside the drape and seals the drape using the ties. A second drape should then be opened, and the drape containing the heart should be placed in the second drape. The heart is then placed into a sterile plastic bag. Alternatively the heart may be transported in a sterile transport solution.

The bag should then be sealed using the heat sealer, making sure it is sealed all the way across twice. The bag should then be placed into an insulated box with wet ice.

Contraindications for cardiac tissue donations are summarised in Table 5.

Table 5. Contraindications for Cardiac Tissue Donation

Factor	Indicator
Time limits	Retrieved up to 48 hours post asystole
Specific	Presence of: • History of, or current malignancy (except treated Carcinoma in situ of the cervix and basal cell carcinoma of the skin); • Sepsis; • Active Multi system auto-immune diseases; • Cardiomyopathy • Endocarditis

19.2.7 Ocular tissue

Criteria for eye donation are summarised in Table 6.

Table 6 Contra indications for eye donation

Criteria	Indicators
Time limits	Retrieved up to 24 hours post asystole
Specific	Leukaemia, lymphomas or myelomas
	Malignant intra-ocular tumours
	Scaring or corneal ulceration
	Corneal laser refractive surgery
	NB – Poor eyesight is not a contraindication to eye donation

19.2.8 Retrieval of Eyes

The whole eye is enucleated. The donor's appearance restored using cotton wool placed in the eye socket, a small plastic disc placed over the cotton wool and the eyelids closed

19.2.9 Retrieval process

Tissue donation after death is performed within a mortuary post-mortem room environment. Ideally this should be dedicated for the purpose. Where this is not possible, donation can take place in other approved environments or operating theatre or in special circumstances (e.g. corneal retrieval) a funeral home. A retrieval organisation may also have their own dedicated donation suite that meets specified room standards.

Time plays a factor in donation, as tissues should be retrieved as soon after death as possible. If the body has not been refrigerated the donation must be completed within 12 hours after death. If the body has been refrigerated within 6 hours of death, donation should preferably start within 24 hours and must be completed within 48 hours of death.

All staff performing tissue donation/retrievals are fully competent and responsible for the procedures they undertake. Full competency and task based training records should be held within their Tissue Establishment.

Prior to the donation procedure, the donor must be prepared in a fashion similar to that of a clinical surgical procedure. All the donation sites are washed and subsequently disinfected. The disinfection process is undertaken by a "sterile" team member to reduce/remove the bacterial load on the surface of the skin. This minimises the bioburden to the donated tissues. Once the retrieval areas have been disinfected, the non-donation sites are then covered using sterile drapes to prevent bacterial contamination to the clean areas.

As with any sterile procedure, a sterile field is prepared away from the donor. The retrieval equipment is placed on the sterile field and can only be used once the retrieval team has donned their sterile clothing, therefore reducing the potential bacterial contamination during the donation process.

As with the consent process, the whole retrieval and donation process is documented within a donor file. This covers the initial retrieval site, health and safety risk assessment, donor identification, donor physical examination and blood/sampling details. This documentation is matched with the consent and medical/behavioural history documentation to provide a complete donation record. This is kept as evidence of the tissue donation and is a legal document.

19.2.10   Donor Identification

Deceased tissue donors must be identified by the person responsible for the retrieval team prior to donation. It is good practice to have this verified by a second team member. The donor must be identified by a minimum of three points of identification; this is imperative to ensure the donation is performed on the consented donor and to ensure the safety of the tissues donated.

Some points of identification that can be used:

- Full name (forename, surname)
- Date of Birth
- Hospital Number
- NHS Number
- Donor Address

19.2.11   Physical examination

Following the identification, a full physical examination is performed looking for any potential medical or behavioural contraindications that may prevent the donation from occurring. These may include (but are not limited to) signs of drug abuse, tattoos/piercings or swellings/ tags.

It is essential that the body of the potential deceased donor has a thorough physical examination prior to the donation commencing. The purpose of the physical examination is to determine donor suitability according to the current standards/legislation and document all findings appropriately.

If there are examples or signs observed during a physical examination or noted in another available record (e.g., hospital records), and are deemed to be an indication of either high risk behaviour or an indication of infections such as HIV or hepatitis, the tissue will be rejected prior to donation.

- Risk of sexually transmitted diseases such as genital ulcerative disease, herpes simplex, syphilis, chancroid and tags, chonylema
- Evidence of non medical percutaneous drug use such as needle marks;
- Needle tracks, including examination of tattoos which may be covering track marks or under the finger/toe nails;
- Unexplained jaundice, or hepatomegaly;
- If the body is rejected for routine post-mortem for infectious criteria or if the post-mortem was undertaken in an infectious control room or under any special precautions and the reasons for these procedures.

Ten important points to remember when performing a physical examination

10   Never believe what someone else tells you;

9   Never take shortcuts;

8   Don't assume a finding means nothing;

7   If you don't know what it is, don't guess;

6   Never be ashamed to ask for help;

5   Always remove all articles of clothing or bandages where possible;

4   Always turn the body over;

3   Inspect all orifices;

2   Describe, don't diagnose;

1   Approach the procedure systematically (i.e. top - bottom, left – right etc).

19.2.12   Considerations when Performing a Physical Examination

General Appearance:
- First impression of the donor;
- Age correlation with description given at referral;
- Height and weight;
- Clothing (if applicable);
- Donor's general hygiene;
- Skin appearance.

Trauma:
- Type and location of injury;
- Direct or indirect impact on donation process;
- Concerns:
  - damage to donated tissue?
  - contamination of tissues?
  - exsanguination.

Skin Interruptions
- Previous injuries/scars;
- Concerns:
  - nature of the injury
  - damage to recovered tissues
  - extent of surgical intervention.

Chronic Conditions/Diseases
- Concerns:
  - Malignancy
  - Infections
  - Systemic disease

19.2.13   Packaging and storage of tissues

All donated tissue are packaged within a double container system at the donation site within the sterile field environment and packaged to defined procedures. All packages are labelled using bar-coding systems as detailed in current guidelines.

Post donation, tissue must be placed at a temperature of 0 - 10°C within 4 hours of retrieval.

19.2.14   Reconstruction

Post donation, the donor is reconstructed to normal anatomical appearance. This is explained during the consent process by the Health Care Professional ensuring the family has complete awareness of how the donor will appear post donation. All incision sites are sutured closed to form a watertight seal and it is essential that seepage is minimised. It is good practice to leave a tag with the donor to provide information regarding the donation with contact details for questions and feedback.

19.3 Blood and Bacteriology sampling

19.3.1 Living Donors

A blood sample must be obtained from the tissue donor. This sample will tested for mandatory blood-borne infections (e.g., Hepatitis B, Hepatitis C) as defined within current guidelines/legislation, additional non-mandatory tests (e.g., malarial antibody test) may be performed if there is evidence from the donor's medical or behavioural history that there is a risk of the graft being infected with a specific transmissible disease that can be detected in the blood.

Note must be taken of the fluids (colloids/ blood/ crystalloids) given to the patient in the 24 hours prior to surgery. This is particularly important where there has been significant blood loss. The tissue establishment must have an algorithm to calculate the extent of plasma dilution which would make the blood sample unsuitable for testing.

19.3.2 Bacteriology Sample (surgical bone donation only)

The bone chips taken at the point of donation are placed into two broths – Tryptic Soy Broth and a Thioglycollate Broth. One broth contains a media environment for aerobic bacteria and the other anaerobic bacteria. The broths may be validated to be frozen for up to 3 months prior to sending to the laboratory for incubation.

The broths are incubated for 7 days and a report is issued for each donation. Any growth detected in the broth determines the fate of the donation which is then terminally sterilised.

NB Amniotic Membrane and Heart Valve donation bacteriology samples are taken during the processing session. See Chapter 16.

19.3.3 Deceased Donors

A blood sample must be obtained from a deceased tissue donor. This sample will tested for mandatory blood-borne infections (e.g., Hepatitis B, Hepatitis C) as defined within current guidelines/legislation, additional non-mandatory tests (e.g., Malarial Antibody test) may be performed if there is evidence from the deceased donor's medical or behavioural history that there is a risk of the graft being infected with a specific transmissible disease that can be detected in the blood or the tissues to be grafted.

Blood samples will be preferably taken pre-mortem, not more than 7 days before death. If a pre-mortem sample cannot be obtained, a post-mortem sample must be taken within 24 hours of death. Where a sample is taken post-mortem, it is important the sample is taken away from any intravenous sites where fluids may have been given. This prevents any risk of dilution or contamination of the blood sample.

All blood samples must be labelled with a minimum three points of identification. This identification is imperative to ensure the safety of the tissues donated from the donor for all the potential recipients. Depending upon circumstances, it is possible to use DNA profiling as an alternative point of identification where a second sample (blood/bone marrow) has been obtained during the donation process by the retrieval team. Where this is used, two other points of identification must have been provided on the original sample.

Note must be taken of the fluids (colloids/ blood/ crystalloids) given to the patient in the 24 hours prior to death. This is particularly important where there has been significant blood loss. The tissue establishment must have an algorithm to calculate the extent of plasma dilution which would make the blood sample unsuitable for testing.

19.4 Suggested Reading

1. www.dermatology.co.uk
2. Human Tissue Act (2004). http://www.opsi.gov.uk/acts/acts2004/20040030.htm
3. Guidelines for the Blood Transfusion Services in the United Kingdom (The Red Book) http://www.transfusionguidelines.org.uk/
4. EU Directive for Cells and Tissues (2004/23/EC)
5. Tissue and Cell Donation: An Essential Guide. Dr Ruth Warwick, Dr Deirdre Fehily, Ted Eastlund and Scott Brubaker
6. Tissue Donor Selection Guidelines (www.transfusionguidelines.org.uk)
7. Physical Examination of the potential tissue donor, what does the literature tell us? Beele, H. Wijk, M.V. Bokhorst, A. Geyt, C.V; Cell Tissue Bank (2009) 10: 253-257
8. Human Tissue Authority Directions (www.hta.gov.uk)

19.5 Self Assessment Questions

Multiple Choice Questions

1. What tissues can a living donor donate?

    a. Bone only

    b. Bone, skin and corneas (eyes)

    c. Bone and placenta (amniotic membrane)

    d. Tendons

    e. Corneas only

2. What are the time restrictions for deceased tissue donation?

    a. Tissue must be donated within 48 hours

    b. Tissue must be donated within 72 hours

    c. Tissue must be donated within 48 hours providing the donor has been refrigerated within 6 hours

    d. Tissue must be donated within 12 hours if the donor has not been refrigerated within 6 hours

    e. Tissue must be donated within 6 hours

3. What are the time restrictions for deceased donor blood samples?

    a. Blood samples taken up to 7 days pre-mortem can be used

    b. Blood samples can be collected up to 48 hours post-mortem

    c. Only pre-mortem samples can be used

    d. Blood samples must be collected with 24 hours post-mortem

    e. There are no time restrictions providing all relevant tests can be performed on the samples collected.

4. Why is the deceased tissue donor prepared in a fashion similar to a clinical surgical procedure?

    a. To minimise the bioburden of the donated tissues

    b. To clean the donor

    c. To reduce/remove bacterial load on the skin surface

    d. To comply with a Hospital's or Family's request

    e. To ensure that all recovered tissues are sterile

Short Answer Questions

1. Why is a physical examination performed on a deceased tissue donor? Give examples of evidence that should be sought.

2. How many points of identification are required to identify a deceased tissue donor? Give examples.

Assignments

1. Compare and contrast the consent process between a living and deceased donor making reference to the legislation involved.

2. Describe the actions taken within the deceased tissue retrieval process to ensure the quality and safety of tissue products.

20 TISSUE PROCESSING, STORAGE AND ISSUE

20.1 Introduction

Retrieved tissue has to undergo a number of processing steps to prepare it for its clinical application. A requirement of tissue processing is that it is carried out in a cleanroom environment. The grade of cleanroom is defined by whether the end product is to be terminally sterilised or not.

Tissue processing must be carried out under strict GMP (Good Manufacturing Practice). Processing protocols must be justified by reference to internal validation reports, evidence in the literature and basic scientific principles. General principles set out in the 'Guidelines for the Blood Transfusion Services in the UK' state the following,

- Tissue Banks should have dedicated processing and storage facilities designed and operated to prevent contamination, cross contamination, mislabelling and deterioration of tissues.

- All processes and equipment which affect the safety or quality of tissues must be validated.

- Processing must not change the physical properties of the tissue so as to make them unacceptable for clinical use. Processing steps must be validated to demonstrate that the final product does not have any clinically significant residual toxicity.

The five main groups of tissues retrieved and processed for transplantation (excluding stem cells) are;

- Bone
- Tendons
- Skin
- Heart Valves
- Corneas

20.2 Bone

Bone processing has five main steps.

1. Dissection - bone is dissected removing all of the soft tissue (Figure 1);
2. Cutting / Grinding - bone is cut and ground to required specifications (Figure 2);
3. Washing (see below);
4. Freeze drying - bone is freeze dried to remove sufficient water to allow storage at room temperature (Figure 3);
5. Terminal sterilisation - bone is sterilised by exposure to gamma irradiation to a dose of 25 – 40 Kgy

Figure 1. Bone is dissected to remove the soft tissue

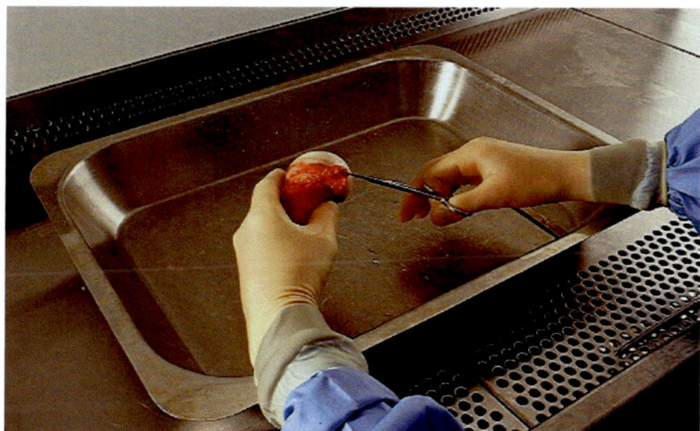

Figure 2. Bone is cut and ground to required specifications

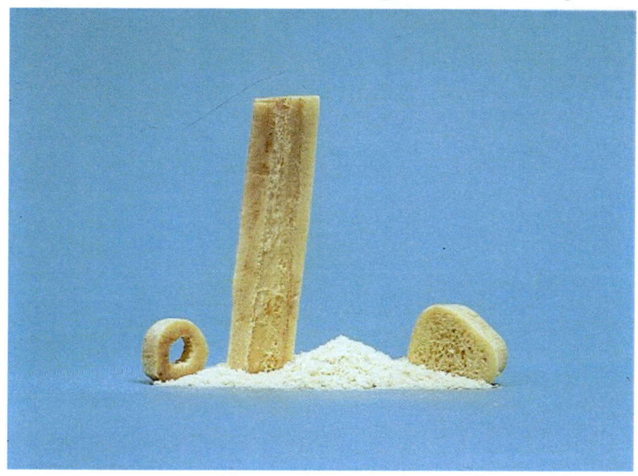

20.2.1 Washing

The purpose of the washing procedure is to remove as much of the blood, marrow and lipid content as possible. There are four reasons for removing this content from bone grafts:

- Removal of the marrow component of the graft has been shown to increase the rate of incorporation *in vivo*;
- There is a possibility that disease causing prions (for example variant CJD) could be present in bone marrow;
- To permit storage at room temperature following lyophilisation. If large amounts of fat are still present, lipid peroxidation occurs and the fat becomes rancid;
- To improve the cosmetic appearance of the graft.

The washing process consists of sonication, pre-centrifuge washing, centrifugation, warm water washing and chemical washing (Table 1).

Table 1. The Washing Process

Step	Detail
Sonication	This is carried out to loosen and disrupt the marrow prior to warm water washing.
Pre-centrifuge washing (50-60°C)	Its main purpose is to melt lipids to ensure their removal during the centrifugation step and to also reduce microbial load.
Centrifugation	The centrifugation process is incorporated to remove primarily the fatty marrow component from large cortico-cancellous grafts and femoral heads.
Warm water washing (50-60°C)	The repeated warm water washing is carried out to reduce microbial load.
Chemical washing	This procedure is carried out to remove marrow components from grafts. Additionally, the chemicals used for this process have known anti-microbial effects.

Figure 3. The Virtis Advantage Freeze Drier

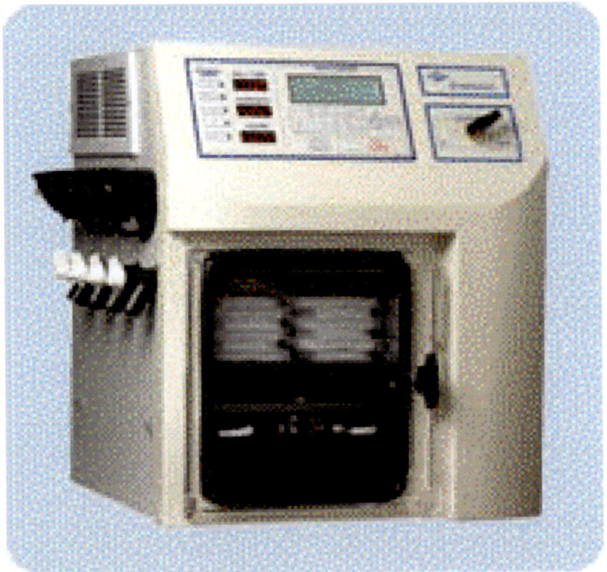

20.3 Tendons

Tendons may be decontaminated or irradiated. Decontaminated tendons are treated with chemicals which remove (if bacteriologically acceptable) the requirement for terminal sterilisation. Irradiated tendons follow the same processing steps as decontaminated tendons but where the bacteriology assessment indicates that the tendon is not suitable as a decontaminated product, the tendon is then sterilised.

Terminally sterilised tendons are a bi-product of decontaminated tendons that have not had their microbial load reduced to a level that does not require sterilisation. As terminally sterilised tendons are initially processed to be decontaminated tendons they must be processed in a cleanroom of a suitable grade for aseptic non-terminally sterilised products.

Tendon processing has four main steps:
- Dissection;
- Cutting;
- Decontamination;
- Terminal sterilisation.

20.3.1 Dissection

Tendons are dissected to remove surrounding soft tissue and cartilage from bone blocks. The side of the tendons are also trimmed to provide clean edges. The tendons are placed in a sterile plastic bag (Figure 4) which is then sealed using a heat sealer, making sure it is sealed all the way across twice. This is then placed inside a secondary bag, and sealed as before using the heat sealer.

Figure 4. Achilles tendon after retrieval

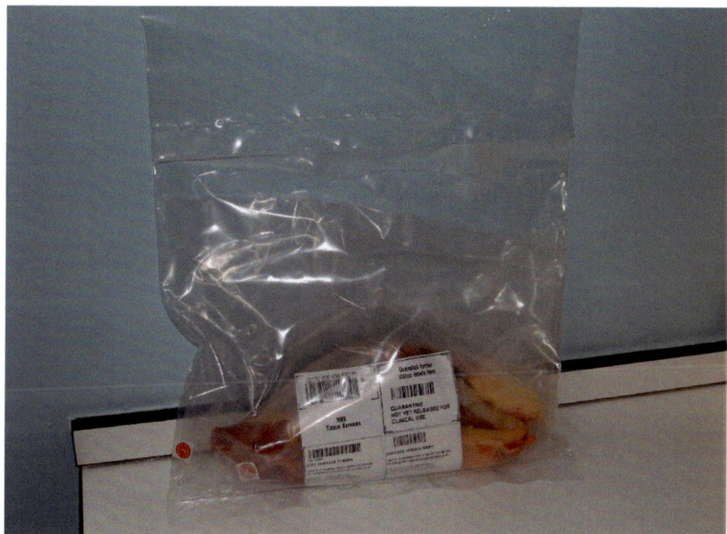

20.3.2 Decontamination

Tendons are decontaminated to reduce the bioburden of the tendon to a level that removes the need for the tendon to be terminally sterilised. The decontamination process consists of a primary decontamination wash, a water wash and a post decontamination bacteriological assessment (Table 2).

Table 2. The Decontamination Process

Step	Detail
Primary decontamination wash (with ethanol)	This is carried out to reduce the microbial load in the tendons.
Water wash	This is carried out to remove any residual alcohol from the decontamination wash.
Post decontamination Bacteriology Sampling	This is carried out assess the microbial load which will determine whether the tendon requires terminal sterilisation.

20.3.3 Terminal Sterilisation

If following decontamination and bacteriological assessment the microbial load is deemed too high the tendon may be suitable for terminal sterilisation. Tendons are terminally sterilised via exposure to Gamma irradiation to a dose of between 25 – 40KGy.

20.4 Skin

20.4.1 Skin Processing

Skin retrieved from deceased donors is not routinely terminally sterilised and therefore should be processed in a suitable grade cleanroom for aseptic products.

Skin, like decontaminated tendons can be terminally sterilised if bacteriological analysis does not permit it to be released as a cryopreserved allograft.

Fundamentally skin is cryopreserved and then stored in liquid nitrogen. There are six main steps to processing skin.

Skin is processed using the following procedure (Figure 5):

1. Bacteriological assessment;
2. Antibiotic treatment - the skin is placed in an antibiotic cocktail and after a series of rinse washes is spread out on gauze;
3. Rinse, size, shape (and bacteriological assessment);
4. Addition of cryoprotectant;
5. Pack;
6. Cryopreserve.

Figure 5. Skin Processing

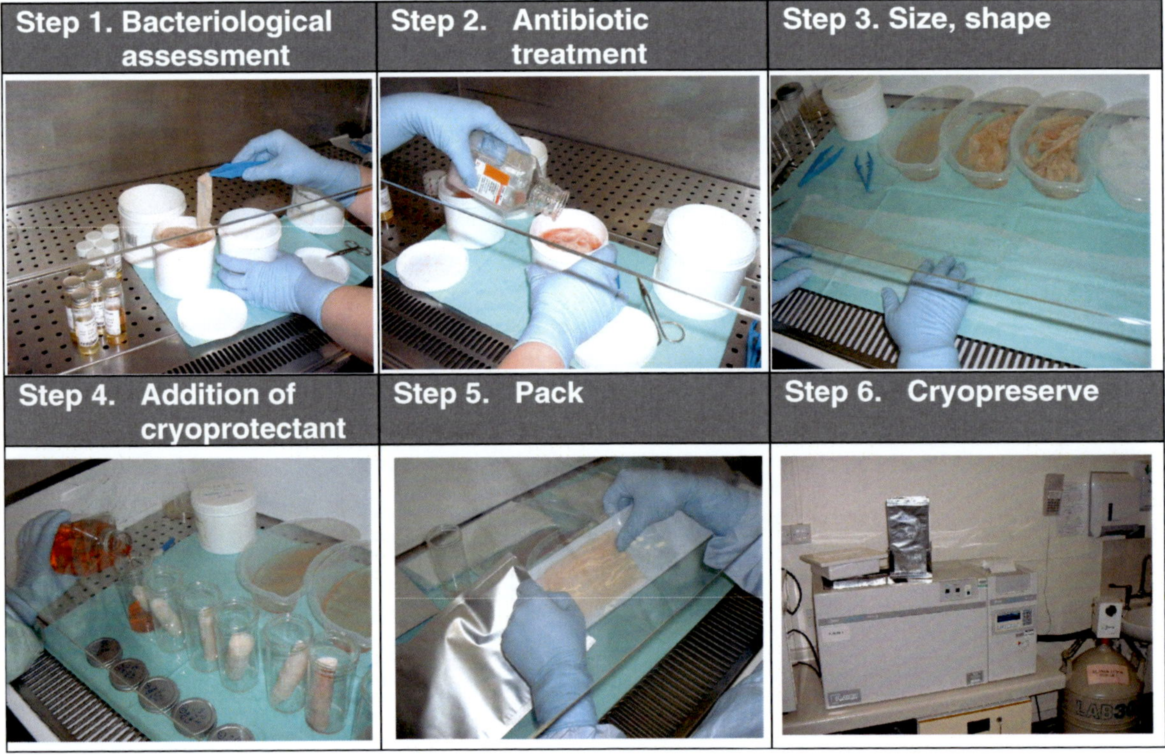

20.5 Heart Valves

20.5.1 Heart Valve Processing

Heart valves cannot be terminally sterilised and therefore have to be processed in a suitable grade cleanroom for aseptic products. Most heart valves are removed from deceased donors but some banks also take the valves from the hearts removed from heart transplant recipients.

Heart valves are processed in the following order (Figure 6):

Figure 6. Heart valve processing

Description	Step
The whole heart is removed in the mortuary or operating theatre.	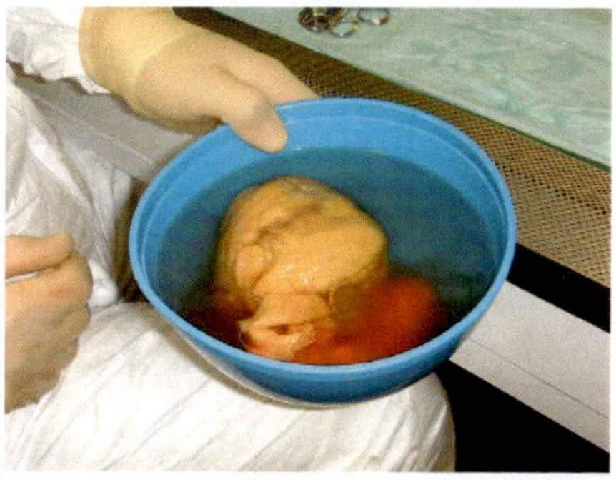
Pulmonary and aortic valves must be dissected from the heart within 72 hours of asystole, the heart having been retrieved from deceased within 48 hours.	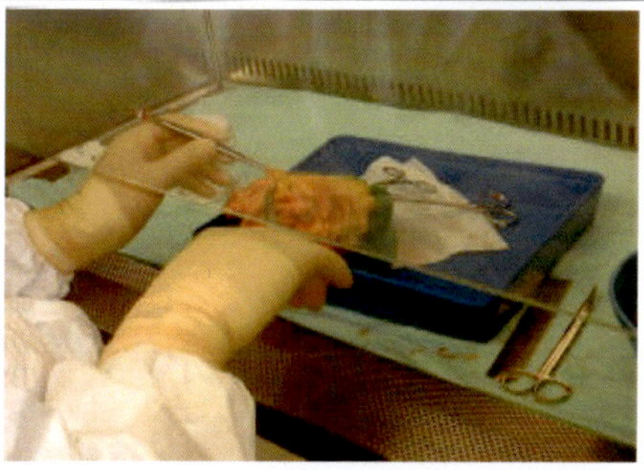
Valve competence and quality assessed at time of dissection	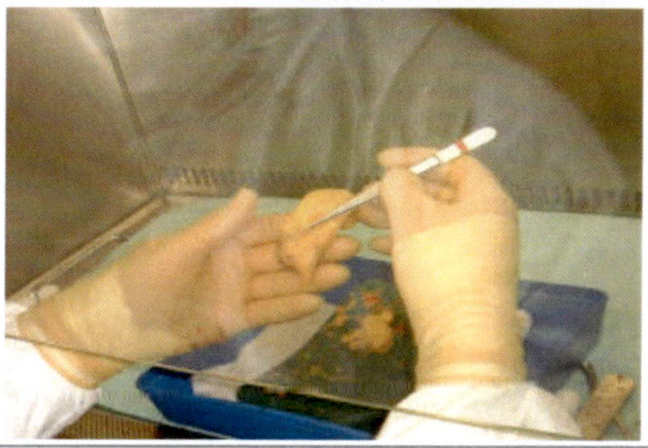

Figure 6. Heart valve processing continued

Description	Step
Heart valve diameter and length are measured.	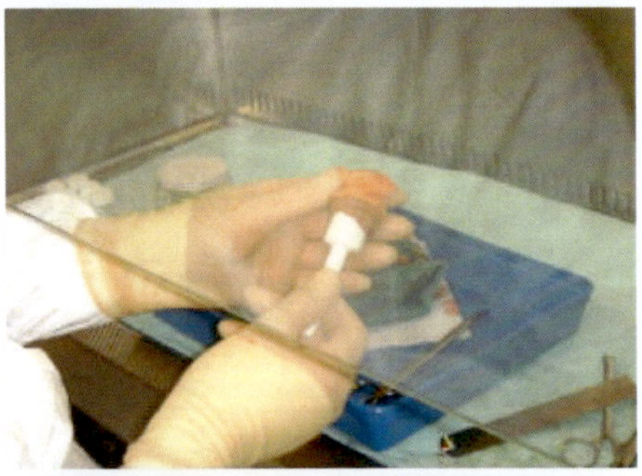 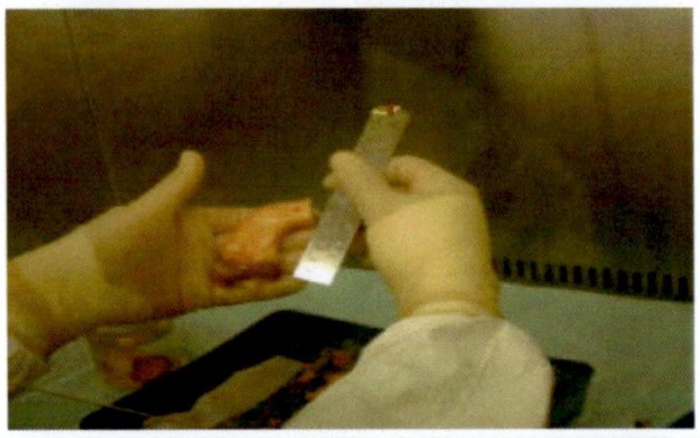
Heart valves are placed in antibiotic solution.	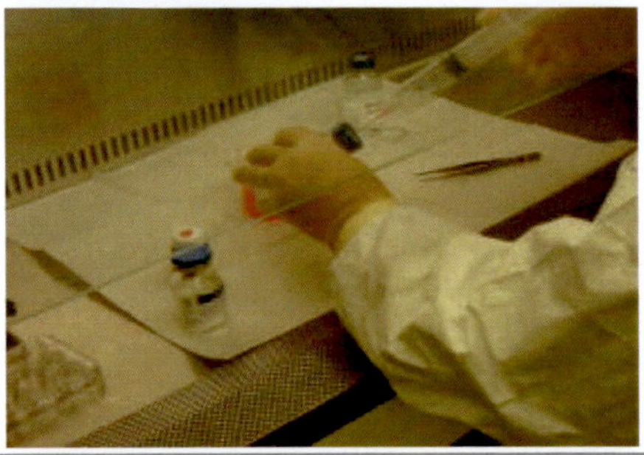
Tissue pieces are tested twice during processing to identify bacterial/fungal contamination.	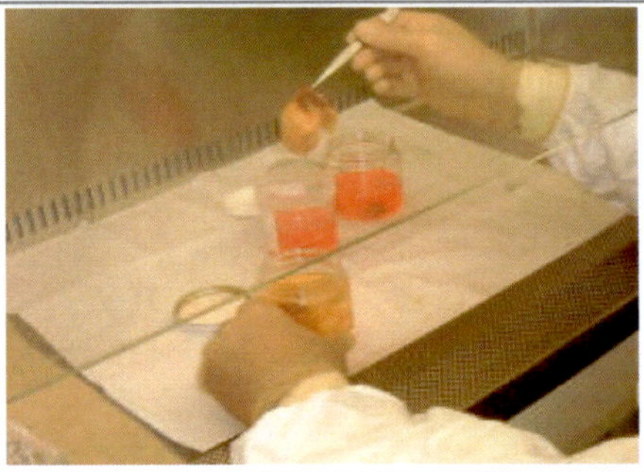

Figure 6. Heart valve processing continued

Description	Step
Heart valves are placed in cryoprotectant fluid and frozen by cooling at a controlled rate of 1°C/min to -110°C. Valves are stored cryopreserved below -140°C for up to 10 years	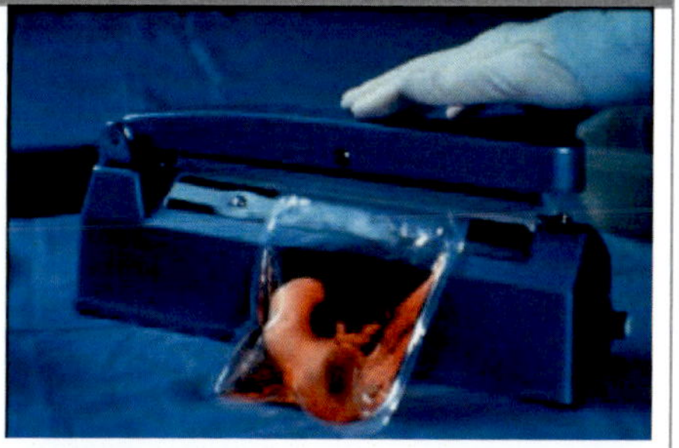 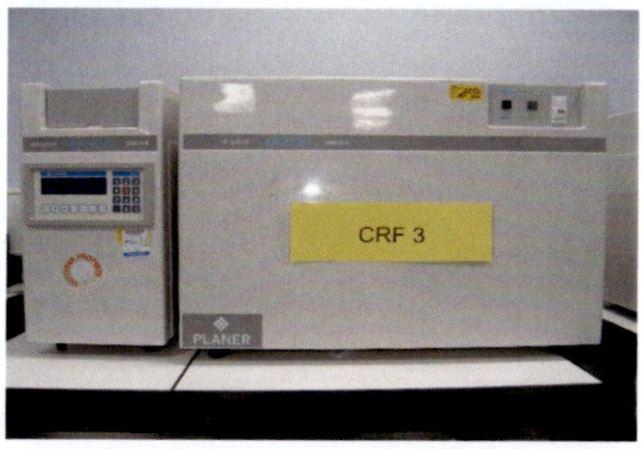 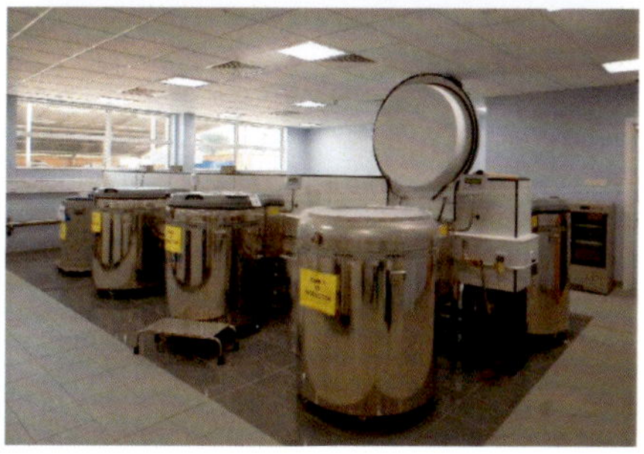

177

20.6 Eyes

20.6.1 Organ culture

Corneas can be stored by organ culture. Eyes are cleaned and corneoscleral disc excised (Figure 7). Corneas are suspended in organ culture medium and then placed in an incubator at 34°C. After 7 days a sample of medium is taken for bacterial/fungal contamination.

Figure 7. Culture of Ocular Tissue

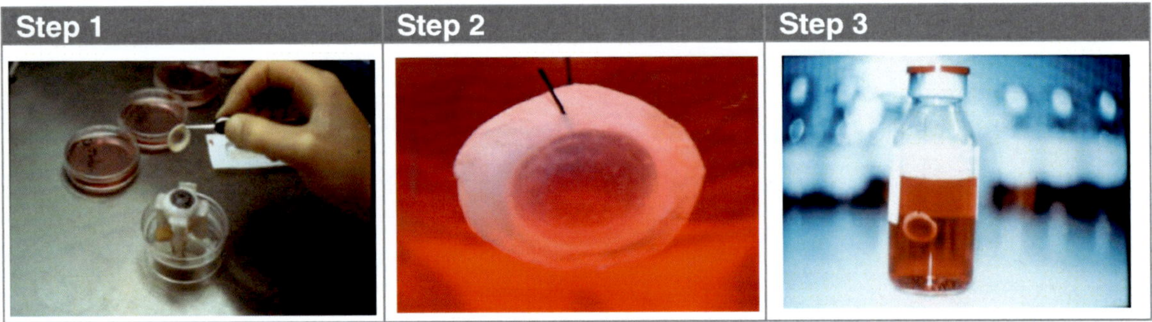

20.6.2 Storage

Storage of corneas:
- Organ culture (34°C) for up to 4 weeks.
- 4°C for 7-10 days.

Storage of sclera:
- 70% ethanol for up to 1 year.

20.6.3 Issuing Corneas for transplantation

Three days before scheduled date of graft, corneal endothelium is examined microscopically. There needs to be a minimum of 2200 cells/mm² to be suitable for transplant. If suitable for transplant, the cornea is placed into medium and returned to 34°C. A sample of medium taken the next day to test for bacteria/fungi. Corneas are despatched at ambient temperature to recipient hospital, the day before the transplant.

20.7 Corneal Storage and Eye Banking

The first eye bank in the USA was opened in New York in 1944 by Richard Townley Paton. Whole eyes were stored in moist chambers at hypothermia and the corneas had to be transplanted within 24-48 hours. This methodology was similar to that introduced by Filatov in the 1930s and it changed little until the 1960s and 1970s when new storage methods were introduced. Independently in the USA and UK, two methods of cryopreservation were developed and some successful corneal transplants were carried out with cryopreserved corneas. Although cryopreservation is the only technique that offers the prospect of truly long-term storage, the complexity and unreliability of the methods, particularly in preserving intact the endothelial layer, meant that they never became part of routine eye bank practice. Today, a very few eye banks keep some cryopreserved corneas for emergency grafts or for partial thickness (lamellar) grafts that do not require living cells.

20.7.1 Hypothermia

Removal of the cornea with a rim of sclera (corneoscleral disc) and storage at 4°C in tissue culture medium containing 5% dextran (McCarey-Kaufman or M-K medium) was introduced in the early 1970s. This increased the storage time for corneas to several days, in part because the corneal endothelium was no longer exposed to deleterious post-mortem changes in the composition of the aqueous humour. This method became widespread because of its simplicity and the medium was also straightforward to make and inexpensive. Even though improved media with extended storage times are now available, M-K medium is still used very successfully by some eye banks, especially in the developing world. One of the improvements was the substitution of much of the dextran by chondroitin sulphate, a glycosaminoglycan found naturally in the corneal stroma. This solution, Optisol-GS, also contained other supplements including vitamins and ATP precursors. Optisol-GS is currently used by the great majority of eye banks in North America. Although corneas can be stored for up to 14 days, the endothelium is better preserved than the epithelium, and most eye banks store corneas in Optisol-GS for no more than 7-10 days.

The benefits of hypothermia derive from the slowing of metabolism in lower temperatures, allowing cells and tissue to survive for longer on limited resources of metabolic substrates. However, cold does not completely suppress metabolism and the reduced capacity for cells to regenerate ATP cannot keep pace with the albeit reduced metabolic demand for energy. With the suppression of active transport of ions, cells gain sodium and lose potassium and because of the fixed negative intracellular charge the Gibbs-Donnan equilibrium means that cells take up water and become oedematous. Calcium homeostasis is also disrupted and cellular acidosis develops. These and other factors serve to limit hypothermic storage times. Other corneal storage media have been devised to address some of these limitations, including Chen medium which aims to support corneal metabolism and a medium that uses Poloxamer 188 (Pluronic F-68) to control stromal oedema instead of chondroitin sulphate or dextran. Poloxamer has been shown to promote cell membrane repair.

20.7.2 Organ Culture

At around the same time as M-K medium was being introduced for hypothermic storage, organ culture methods developed for skin were being applied to cornea. Unlike hypothermic storage, the aim of organ culture was to maintain tissues in near physiological conditions and to support metabolism by supplying nutrients. A major advantage of organ culture was that it extended the storage time from just a few days to four weeks.

Despite this, it was thought in the USA to be overly complicated and the corneas were considered to be overly prone to bacterial and fungal contamination. There was also difficulty in trying to reverse the significant stromal oedema that occurred during organ culture storage. Attempts to reverse the oedema by placing the corneas in M-K medium at 4°C prior to transplantation resulted in increased post-operative loss of endothelial cells. In Europe, however, these problems were later solved and organ culture became an established method in most of the major European eye banks and is also used in the Auckland Eye Bank in New Zealand. Paradoxically, the microbiological contamination issue that caused such concern in the USA came to be seen as an advantage since it meant that by routine monitoring of the organ culture medium during corneal storage there was a greater chance of detecting corneas infected by bacteria and fungi, thereby preventing their transplantation. Moreover, an integral part of the organ culture method is a cleaning protocol for the ocular surface before excision of corneoscleral discs in order to reduce microbial contamination (e.g., several rinses in sterile saline and immersion in 1-3% Povidone-iodine).

During organ culture, antibiotics and antimycotics are far more effective against bacteria and fungi than the antibiotics in hypothermic storage media owing to the higher temperature.

Typical organ culture conditions use a medium such as Eagle's Minimum Essential Medium (although other basal media are also used) containing 2-8% serum and antibiotics/antimycotic with corneas being stored at 31-34°C. A few eye banks store corneas at 37°C, but this is in fact slightly higher than physiological temperature for corneas, which is closer to 34°C. Most eye banks keep corneas under these conditions for up to 4 weeks, although corneas have been successfully transplanted after 7 weeks in organ culture. Some eye banks change the medium at weekly intervals, whereas others do not change the medium. To a certain extent, this depends on the volume of medium, which may be up to 80 ml in a glass DIN bottle with the cornea suspended in the medium by a suture through the scleral rim. Plastic tissue culture flasks are also used. The stromal oedema is reversed by placing the corneas into medium containing 5% dextran and keeping them at organ culture temperature. The corneas also tolerate storage at ambient temperature in this medium for 3-4 days, facilitating transport from the eye bank to hospitals. Poloxamer and hydroxyethyl starch have also been used for thinning corneas before transplantation.

20.7.3 Endothelial Assessment

Since the successful outcome of a corneal transplant is heavily dependent on the donor endothelium, an important part of the process is the examination of the corneal endothelium by light microscopy. This allows an estimate of endothelial cell density, most eye banks setting a minimum cell density of 2000-2500 cells/mm², and to check for areas of cell loss or damage. In the organ culture technique, a typical method of endothelial examination involves staining with trypan blue to detect damaged cells and use of hypo-osmotic saline or sucrose to render the endothelial cell borders visible under transmitted light or phase-contrast microscopy. As endothelial cell density declines with age, the numbers of corneas not meeting the minimum cell density understandably increases with increasing donor age. While approximately 80% of corneas from donors under 60 years old exceed the minimum cell density, only 50% of corneas from donors older than 80 years do so. However, this means that many corneas from these older donors are suitable for transplantation. Despite this, some eye banks, especially in North America, still set upper age limits for eye donors. Based on modelling of endothelial cell loss in corneal transplants, it has been estimated that if corneal transplants survive the initial 3-4 years, during which they are most prone to complications and rejection, they are likely to survive for at least 25 years before the endothelial cell density falls to a level where the endothelium is no longer able to maintain corneal transparency.

In UK there is no upper age limit for corneal donation, but the issue of lower endothelial density in older donors is addressed by donor recipient age matching namely the age difference should not be greater than 20 years.

20.7.4 Donor Selection Criteria

In general, many eye donor exclusion criteria are in common with criteria for other cells and tissues. Standard serological markers of transmissible disease are screened and degenerative neurological conditions, death from unknown cause, and a number of specific systemic or ocular diseases or infections are contraindications to transplantation of ocular tissue. However, a major divergence in the selection criteria compared with other cells and tissues is the acceptance of donors with solid tumours. Haematological neoplasms are excluded as are malignant tumours in the anterior segment of the eye and retinoblastoma.

This is again down to the avascular nature of the cornea. Since sclera and limbal tissue are vascularised tissues, the use of these tissues from donors with solid tumours is contraindicated.

20.8 Suggested Reading

1. Kearney JN. Guidelines on processing and clinical use of skin allografts. Clin Dermatol. 2:357-364 (2005)

2. Kearney J N. Quality issues in skin banking: a review. Burns. 24:299-305 (1998)

3. Fehily D and Warwick R. Tissue Banking. In *Practical Transfusion Medicine.* (Eds M Murphy and D Pamphilon). Pp 317-326

4. Kearney J.N. Banking of skin grafts and biological dressings. In *Principles and Practice of Burns Management* (Ed JAD Settle). Pp329-351.

5. Tissue banking: tissue retrieval and processing. In *Guidelines for the Blood Transfusion Service in the United Kingdom.* Chapter 23, 7th Edition.

6. Rules and Guidance for Pharmaceutical Manufacturers and Distributors (2002) Annex 1; Manufacture of Sterile Medicinal Products.

7. Code of Practice (5): The Removal, Storage and Disposal of Human Organs and Tissue. Human Tissue Authority.

20.9 Self Assessment Questions

Multiple Choice Questions

1. What is the required irradiation dose of gamma irradiation for tissue sterilisation?
    a) 20 – 35 kGy
    b) 25 – 40 kGy
    c) 25 – 45 kGy
    d) 30 – 40 kGy
    e) 45 – 55 kGy

2. Tendons are decontaminated using which of the following?
    a) Hydrogen peroxide
    b) Klericide
    c) Sodium chloride
    d) Ethanol
    e) Gamma irradiation

3. What temperature are heart valves cryopreserved to, prior to storage?
    a) -10°C
    b) -135°C
    c) -40°C
    d) -80°C
    e) 4°C

4. Which of the following statements is false?
    a) The grade of cleanroom used for processing is defined by whether the end product is terminally sterilised or not.
    b) Processing must not change the physical properties of the tissue.
    c) All processes which affect the safety and quality of tissues must be validated.
    d) Only tissues that fail bacteriology testing need to be sterilised.
    e) The majority of corneas are stored by organ culture.

5. What is the typical maximum storage time for corneas in organ culture?
    a) 1 week
    b) 2 weeks
    c) 4 weeks
    d) 6 weeks
    e) 8 weeks

6. What is most widely used hypothermic storage medium in North America?
    a) Optisol-GS
    a) Chen Medium
    b) M-K medium
    c) Eagle's MEM
    d) RPMI

1. The purpose of washing bone is to remove as much of the blood, marrow and lipid content as possible. What are the four reasons for removing this content from bone grafts?

2. Why and how are tendons decontaminated?

3. Why is organ culture thought to improve the microbiological safety of corneal transplants compared with hypothermic storage?

Assignments

1. Discuss the role of Good Manufacturing Practice (GMP) in assuring the quality and safety of processed tissues for transplantation.

2. Bone processing involves dissection, cutting, washing, freeze drying and sterilisation. What are the purposes of these steps and how would the failure of a step effect the end product?

3. Discuss the advantages and disadvantages of organ culture vs. hypothermic storage of corneas.

21 CLINICAL ASPECTS OF TISSUE TRANSPLANTATION

21.1 Introduction

Tissues like skin, bone, tendons, heart valves and cornea are used in surgical procedures to replace lost or damaged tissues in the patients. The source of such tissues (grafts) can be from another part of the body of the same individual, from another person or another species to serve as replacement (Table 1). There are also synthetic alternatives.

Table 1. Classification of Grafts

Graft	Source
Autograft	Tissue from same individual
Allograft	Tissue from another individual of the same species
Xenograft	Tissue from another species
Synthetic graft	Implants made of synthetic materials

Currently donated tissue allografts have an important role in enhancing the quality of life of the recipients. Some examples and uses of tissue allografts are given in Table 2 and are discussed in more detail below. The advances in the field of science have opened opportunities for new bio-engineered products in regenerative medicine. The safety and efficacy these new methods have to be clinically evaluated by structured randomised controlled trials to determine their role in treating patients in the future.

Table 2. Tissue Products and Their Clinical Use

Tissue Products	Common Surgical Procedures
Frozen Femoral Head	Impaction grafting in joint revision surgery
Cancellous bone chips	Non union of fracture
Cortical bone struts and rings	Spinal disc surgery
Demineralised bone	Dental and maxillofacial surgery
Distal femur, proximal tibia etc., (massive bone allograft)	Reconstruction after surgery for bone tumour
Tendons	Reconstruction of knee ligaments
Aortic and Pulmonary valves	Replace damaged or diseased valves
Skin	Temporary dressing in major burns
Cornea	To replace diseased or damaged corneas
Amniotic membrane	Reconstruction of ocular surface

21.2 Diseases Treated with Cardiovascular Grafts

Human heart valves have been successfully implanted since the 1960s. The past fifty years have seen continued improvements in cryopreservation methods and surgical procedures and these have been associated with improved clinical outcome. The heart is retrieved from deceased donors and aseptically processed into aortic and pulmonary valves or non-valve conduits. The alternatives to cryopreserved human heart valves are mechanical heart valves and porcine (pig) heart valves. The implantation of the allograft is technically more challenging for the surgeon than other types of valves. The distinct advantages of using cryopreserved human heart valves are lower incidence of calcification and infection and, hence reduced chances of re-operation over the long term. Moreover, patients do not require long term anticoagulation therapy unlike those with mechanical valve replacement.   The availability of allograft especially smaller sizes is restricted by limited donor availability.

Processed femoral vein has been used in patients requiring vascular reconstruction. This is particularly useful in access surgery for patients requiring arteriovenous shunts. In addition arterial grafts are used to replace infected prosthetic grafts.

21.3 Diseases Treated with Musculoskeletal Grafts and Implants

21.3.1 Bone Grafts

Musculoskeletal products are used in a wide variety of surgical procedures ranging from joint replacement in old age to sports injuries in the young. Bone is most often used in impaction grafting procedures in revision hip surgery, i.e. when a primary hip replacement has failed and a new prosthesis has to be used to replace the bone removed during the first operation. The purpose of bone grafting is to provide "linkage", like filling bony cavities or defects or "splintage" for treatment of ununited fracture as well to promote osteogenesis.

<u>Autologous</u> bone is the best graft material because it does not carry the risk of viral infection although it can become bacterially infected. The bone is mostly harvested from iliac crest or from proximal tibia and distal radius. The cancellous bone can be used to fill bony defects and cortical bone is used to provide structural support. The grafted bone forms a scaffold into which osteoblasts and osteocasts can grow. The osteoblasts lead to graft resorption and the mediators released during this process (osteoinduction) stimulate local bone growth. The use of autograft is limited by bone availability and may not be suitable to fill massive segmental bone loss. The autograft is also not suitable in areas of significant load bearing. Surgically it carries a disadvantage of increased morbidity because it requires extra operative time to harvest associated with a longer anaesthetic and, in addition, the patient will have two operation sites rather than one.

<u>Allogeneic</u> bone is more plentiful and harvested from living donors (following hip replacement) or from deceased donors. Allograft bone is available as:

- Demineralised bone matrix –used primarily for dental and maxillofacial surgery
- Morsellised bone for impaction grafting
- Strut and ring grafts to cover cortical bone
- Massive allografts to replace significant portion of native bone

Infection is the major concern with allografts and bacteria can be eliminated with irradiation of the graft or by other validated chemical procedures.

<u>Bone substitutes</u>: There is interest in artificial bone substitute, as this would eliminate supply and infection problems associated with auto and allografts. Possible bone substitutes include calcium triphosphate, hydroxyapatite and calcium carbonate. Most of the available substitutes are brittle and unable to withstand significant weight bearing.

21.3.2 Tendon and Meniscus Grafts

Tendons are generally used to replace or repair a torn tissue – often the grafted tissue is shaped and not as wide as the original but the strength of the tendon still allows full function of the joint. Tendon grafts are mainly used in the field of sports medicine.   The grafts can be supplied as decontaminated or irradiated tendons. A recently published metanalysis included six studies which compared the allograft and autograft recipients with a minimum of two years follow up. The results indicate that the sterilisation process affects graft quality. There was no difference in the outcome between the allograft and autograft recipients if patients receiving irradiated or chemically processed grafts were excluded from the evaluation of results.

Allograft tendons normally supplied include patellar tendons whole or shaped (BPTB-bone patellar tendon bone), achilles tendon and hamstrings (semitendinosus and gracilis). The patellar tendon can be used for anterior cruciate ligament (ACL) reconstruction and the Achilles tendon can be used for posterior cruciate ligament (PCL) reconstruction.

Tears in menisci occur in the young mainly through sports injuries and in the old through wear and tear. Such tears are treated by meniscectomy. However, the symptoms such as pain and swelling recur years following removal of the damaged meniscus. This progresses to arthritis with further worsening of the symptoms. Meniscal allografts are used in patients who have developed symptoms following previous meniscectomy to prevent long term damage to the joint.

21.4 Diseases Treated with Skin Grafts

Skin grafts are used to cover an area of skin defect that is too large to be treated by direct closure using simple suturing. The skin loss can occur following burns, skin infection, surgery to skin cancer, or from an injury.

The best skin grafts come from the patient's own body (autograft). The graft is taken from another part of body (donor site), and transplanted on to the affected area (recipient site). The skin is made up of two layers: epidermis and dermis. In full thickness graft both layers are included in the graft. As no dermis is left behind at the donor site, the skin will not grow back and the edges of donor site are sutured together for the site to heal. For this reason only small grafts are possible and are normally taken from inner side of upper arm, groin and behind the ears. A partial thickness graft or split skin graft includes epidermis and part of dermis. Donor site can regenerate and can heal in fourteen days.

In the case of burns victims, when the patient does not have enough healthy skin to donate, temporary coverage using allogeneic skin from deceased donors may be used to protect against infection, reduce fluid loss, reduce pain and to allow the tissues underneath to heal. However, the patient's immune system recognises the allograft as foreign material and the graft is rejected in one to three weeks. The graft is then removed.

Though risk of transmission of infection or disease is extremely low due to careful donor selection, testing and validated processing methods, it is a good practice to limit the donor exposure to the recipient, e.g. when a burns victim needs large quantities of skin allografts, the skin packs retrieved from the same donor should be assigned to the recipient.

Donor skin is in short supply to meet the demand. The advances in research in biotechnology have produced new types of skin grafts. The cultured epithelial autograft (CEA) uses living skin cells from the patient to culture sheets of new skin cells in the laboratory. Being an autograft, the graft is not rejected and forms a permanent layer of new skin. The CEA are thin, delicate and fragile and hence patients may need longer hospitalisation to reduce movements till the grafts are established. One of the main issues in using CEA is that it takes time (2-3 weeks) for the epithelial cells to grow and become confluent.

In recent years, several "artificial skin" products have become available which are used as temporary dressing for massive burns. The artificial skin usually consists of a synthetic epidermis and collagen-based dermis, which acts as a template for the formation of new tissue.

Skin is used in the early, life-saving treatment of major burns (Figure 1) as a temporary wound closure graft or biological dressing to:

- Reduce interference with the wound from dressings;
- Stimulate underlying tissues;
- Prepare a good dermal bed for later grafting.

One severely burned patient may need skin from up to five donors.

Figure 1. Allograft Skin for Burns Treatment

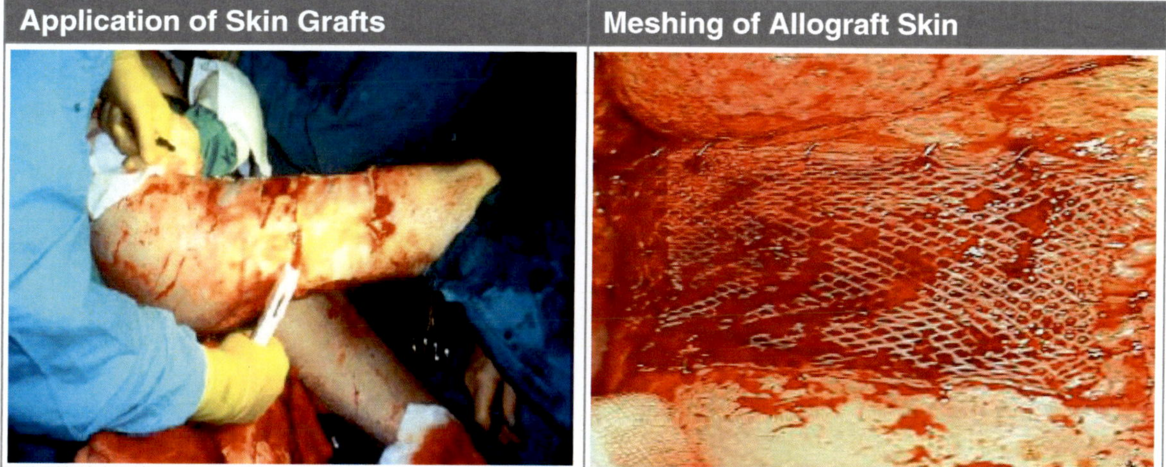

21.5 Ocular Tissue Transplantation

There are several different types of ocular tissue transplants depending on which part of the cornea is damaged or non-functioning through disease of injury.

21.5.1 Penetrating Keratoplasty (PK)

These are full-thickness grafts including all of the layers of the cornea. A disc of diseased cornea, typically 7-7.5 mm in diameter, is removed from the patient's eye using a trephine. This is replaced with a disc of healthy tissue cut from a donor cornea. The graft is sutured in place using extremely fine sutures. Because the cornea is avascular, healing is very slow depending purely on slow migration of cells between graft/ host border, therefore, the sutures can remain in place for up to a year or more. This is currently the most common type of ocular tissue transplant. A healthy endothelium on the donor cornea is essential to the successful outcome of the transplant. Full-thickness graft survival depends mainly on the indication for transplantation.

Despite the lack of blood vessels in normal cornea, corneal transplants are prone to immunological allograft rejection, and rejection is one of the main causes of graft failure. Survival tends to be high in transplants for keratoconus and Fuchs' endothelial dystrophy (>90% at one year). Even after 10 years, survival remains at 90% for keratoconus and 75% for Fuchs'. By contrast, for other corneal diseases, survival can be as low as 60% at one year, falling to 40% at 10 years. Another complication of PK is post-operative astigmatism, where the curvature of the cornea varies in different areas causing distortion of vision.

21.5.2 Lamellar Grafts

Lamellar grafts are partial thickness grafts that do not include all corneal layers. They were first used for replacing anterior stroma but in recent years rapid development in surgical techniques allowed to include deep anterior lamellars (DALK) where virtually the full thickness of the stroma is replaced, leaving the patient's endothelium intact. These are particularly suitable for keratoconus, which is primarily a stromal rather than an endothelial disease. There are also techniques for replacing just the endothelium on a thin strip of stroma, leaving the patient's own stroma intact. These grafts are used where the problem is primarily endothelial disease. A major advantage of these techniques over PK is lesser post operational trauma that allows quick visual recovery; it also helps in reduction of astigmatism.

21.5.3 Limbal Grafts

For patients with ocular surface disease caused by limbal stem cell deficiency, chemical burns to the eye and the other traumas that involve extensive damage to the limbal area; grafts of limbal tissue, sometimes combined with amniotic membrane, can successfully restore the corneal epithelium. An alternative is to grow out the stem cells and expand them ex vivo into cell sheets that can then be transplanted on a fibrin or amniotic membrane carrier.

21.5.4 Sclera

Sclera can be used for coating orbital implants following therapeutic enucleation. It is also used for reconstructive surgery and in certain types of glaucoma surgery.

21.6 Diseases Treated with Ocular or Amniotic Membrane Grafts

The cornea is the clear tissue at the front of the eye that lets in light and helps focus it on the retina. The cornea may become cloudy or distorted in shape either by disease or injury causing loss of vision. Some examples of indications for corneal transplant include:

- Keratoconus, an eye disorder in which the middle of the cornea thins and eventually bulges outward
- Bullous keratopathy, a progressive swelling and blistering of the cornea
- Severe corneal ulcers caused by bacterial, fungal, parasitic or viral eye infections
- Severe traumatic injuries that pierce or cut the cornea
- Chemical burns of the eye
- Corneal scars
- Fuch's endothelial dystrophy, a progressive eye disease that causes swelling, cloudiness and blistering of the cornea
- Failure or rejection of a previous corneal transplant

The first successful corneal transplant was reported in 1905. In the UK, more than 44,000 cornea transplants have been recorded in the National Transplant Database since the corneal transplant service began in 1983.

The amniotic membrane, or amnion, comprises the innermost layer of the placenta. Amniotic membrane transplant (AMT) has been successfully used in a number of procedures for restoration of the ocular surface following chemical, thermal, surgical trauma or severe scarring. Amnion is used because of its ability to diminish the occurrence of adhesions and scarring, its ability to enhance wound healing and its antimicrobial potential. More randomised controlled trials are required to compare the outcome of AMT with other conventional treatment options to determine the safety and efficacy of AMT to treat different ocular conditions.

Approximately 2500 cornea and 200 sclera transplants are conducted each year in the UK. Figure 2 summarises the main clinical indications.

Figure 2. Indications for Corneal Transplantation

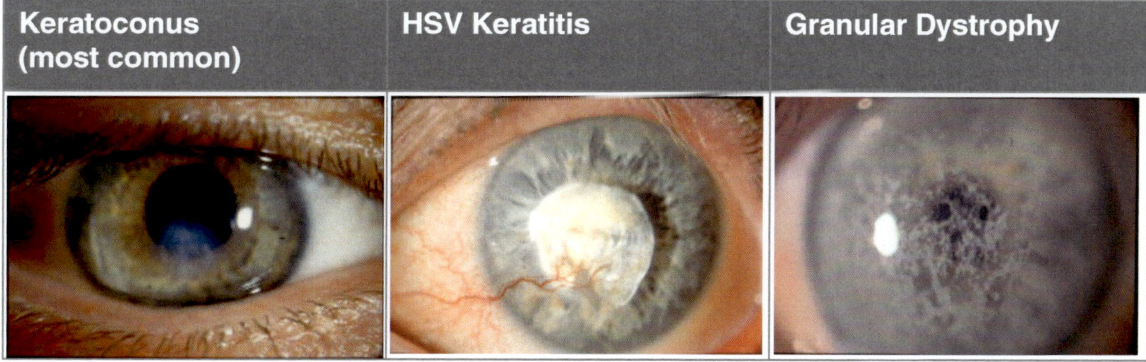

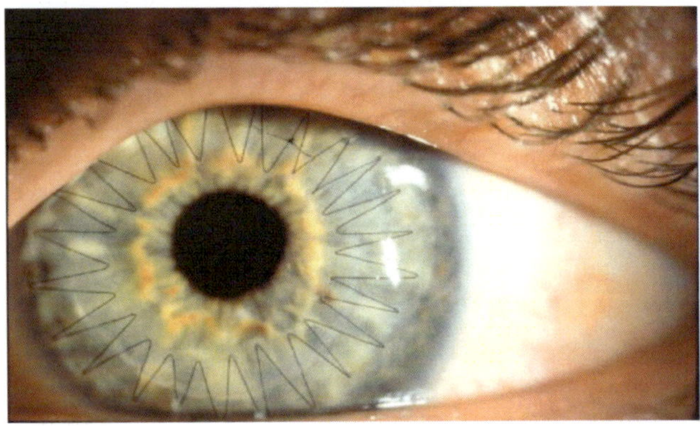

21.7 Diseases that Could be Potentially Treated with Tissue Engineered Products

The principle of tissue engineering (TE) is to use the combination of cell transplantation, material engineering and suitable biochemical factors to improve or restore the biological functions in diseased or injured tissue. Tissue engineered products (TEP) (e.g.: skin, cartilage) are already available for clinical use. The pluripotent stem cells implanted in appropriate location can generate the intended tissues like bone, cartilage or tendon. TE field is still in its infancy. Because of this, the clinical applications are yet to be validated by controlled randomised trials. Other than direct use of tissue engineered products, it is anticipated that TE will have an impact on several other areas of medicine in the future. The ability to understand how cells develop (microenvironment) may lead to scientific advances in defining appropriate therapies.

Under European commission's proposals, the TEP would be regulated under "Advanced Therapy Medicinal Products". A directive has been issued (1394/2007) and is in the process of being implemented.

21.8 Risk Factors in Tissue Transplantation

21.8.1 Infection

In the UK, the tissue donors are selected carefully following national donor selection guidelines. Donors with history of malignancy, diseases of unknown aetiology, neurodegenerative disorders and those with high-risk lifestyle history for transmissible infections like HIV and Hepatitis B or Hepatitis C are excluded from donation. The tissues are retrieved by trained staff using aseptic methods.

All tissue donors are tested for mandatory markers similar to blood donors using validated serological tests to detect specific antibodies (as in the case of HIV and Hepatitis C), antigen tests (as in Hepatitis B) and extremely sensitive nucleic acid testing. (These are described in more detail in Chapter 5). Moreover, due to the retrieval conditions and the amount of complex processing that may be involved in various tissue processes, a significant amount of in-process and end stage bacteriological testing is undertaken. There are well documented cases where fatal bacterial transmissions have taken place with fatal consequences to the recipient.

The range of viral, bacterial and fungal transmissions is wide and therefore utmost care is required to all aspects of tissue donation, from donor medical screening, blood testing, tissue testing and rigorous process controls to minimize these risks.

Table 3. Disease transmitted by tissues

Tissue	HIV	HBV	HCV	HTLV	CMV	CJD	Rabies	Malaria	Bacteria	Fungi	TB
Bone	√		√						√		√
Cornea		√			√	√	√		√	√	
Dura						√					
Heart Valves		√									√
Bone Marrow					√			√			
Skin	√				√				√		
Tendons	√		√								

21.9 Tracking of Tissues and Reporting Adverse Events

The EU Tissues and Cells directive came into force from April 2006, throughout the EU, to create a common framework for ensuring safety and quality of the tissues and cells used for therapeutic purposes. There are two detailed technical annexes to the parent directive. The first was published in February 2006 and, the second in October 2006. The second annex stipulates requirements for traceability of tissues and notification of serious adverse reactions and events.

It is the responsibility of the tissue establishments to maintain records and have policies and procedures in place to investigate or notify any serious adverse events in the donor or the recipient, which may influence the quality or safety of the tissues. Most tissue banks supply tissues directly to the hospital theatre departments. The users should be advised to (a) keep records of receipt of tissues received and their fate (b) to record the donation number of tissue in the recipient's notes, and (c) to inform the tissue bank of any suspected adverse event that might be attributable to the transplanted tissue.

The Human Tissue Authority (HTA) is the competent authority in the UK under the European directive and has the responsibility for licensing and storage of human tissues (excluding gametes). The tissue bank must notify the HTA of any suspected serious adverse reactions or events without any delay.

21.10 Suggested Reading

1. Fehily D and Warwick R. Tissue banking. In, *Practical Transfusion Medicine*. (Eds M Murphy and D Pamphilon, 2nd ed). Blackwell Science. Pp 309-319.

2. Tissue banking: safety of human tissues and cells for transplantation. In, *Future Strategies for Tissue and Organ Replacement*. (Eds. J Polak, L Hench, P Kemp, D Fehily, RM Warwick, JN Kearney). Imperial College Press (London). 2002.

3. Saw VPJ et al. Amniotic membrane transplantation for ocular disease: a prospective evaluation of the first 233 cases from the UK user group. Br J Opthamol. 2007 (in press).

4. Warwick RM et al. The role of the Blood Transfusion Service in Tissue Banking. Vox Sanguinis 71: 71-77 (1996).

5. Fehily D et al. Safe tissue grafts should achieve the same standards as for blood transfusion. BMJ, 314:1141-1142 (1997).

6. Warwick R M et al Tissue and Cell Donation An essential guide. Wiley Blackwell (eds Warwick RM Fehily D Brubaker S and Eastlund T) 2009

7. McDermott ID. What tissue bankers should know about the use of allograft meniscus in orthopaedics. Cell Tissue Bank DOI 10.1007/s 10561-009-9127-2 (Online 2009)

8. Barron DJ, Khan NE et al. What tissue bankers should know about the use of allograft heart valves. Cell Tissue Bank DOI 10.1007/s10561-009-9132-5 (Online 2009)

9. Getgood A, Bollen S. What tissue bankers should know about the use of allograft tendons and cartilage in orthopaedics. Cell Tissue Bank DOI 10.1007/s10561-009-9129-0 (Online 2009)

10. Rauz S, Saw VP. Serum eye drops, amniotic membrane and limbal epithelial cells – tools in the treatment of ocular surface disease. Cell Tissue Bank DOI 10.1007/s10561-009-9128-1(Online 2009)

21.11 Self Assessment Questions

Multiple Choice Questions

1) What is an allograft?
   a) Tissue from same individual
   b) Tissue from another individual of same species
   c) Tissue from another species
   d) Graft made of synthetic materials
   e) Tissue which has been processed

2) Allogeneic skin is used in the treatment of:
   a) Direct closure of skin wound
   b) Surgery for skin cancer
   c) Burns victims
   d) Skin infections
   e) Severe fungal infections

3) Which of the following are true about amniotic membrane transplantation (AMT)?
   a) AMT is used to repair duramater in brain surgery
   b) Amnion is donated by deceased multi-tissue donors
   c) Amnion delays wound healing
   d) AMT may be used to treat ocular scarring
   e) AMT may be used to treat burns

4) The competent authority in the UK for licensing tissue establishments is:
   a) European Commission
   b) Council of Europe
   c) MHRA
   d) HTA
   e) HFEA

Short Answer Questions

1. What are the advantages of cryopreserved human heart valves?
2. What are the risks associated with the use of allografts and what steps can be taken to minimise these adverse effects?

Assignments

1. Describe recent advances in the field of tissue engineering and the potential use of the products in regenerative medicine?
2. What steps can be taken to meet the EU requirement for traceability of donated tissues?

22 TISSUE ENGINEERING

Tissue replacements used in surgery have typically comprised of tissue allografts or animal derived xenografts where the donor tissue has simply been treated to ensure long-term preservation prior to use. The tissues have either been banked as viable (living) grafts, where steps are taken to preserve cell viability, or as non-living grafts. No attempt is made to modify the tissue significantly to enhance incorporation, performance or longevity of the graft.

Although traditional tissue banking has provided important additions to the surgeon's options for treatment, there are certain generic limitations. With non-living tissues there are no viable cells present within the tissue. Unless the patient's (recipient's) cells are able to re-colonise the graft, the long-term consequences are that the graft would be unable to self repair and unable to grow (e.g. when implanted in a child). The latter may therefore necessitate frequent re-operations. Some tissues are readily re-colonised e.g. cancellous bone. Bone has a very high natural turnover rate in the body, so there are natural mechanisms for rapid regeneration. In contrast, other tissues are not readily, if ever, re-colonised, such as blood vessels and heart valves.

This limitation can be overcome by implanting viable grafts. In this case however, the cells are allogeneic in origin and are therefore likely to elicit an immunological rejection response. This response will kill the allogeneic cells, and may cause collateral damage to the graft tissue. There is evidence that the recipient's response to either living cells or dead cells in a graft may inhibit, or at least slow down the re-colonisation process. In addition, preservation of <u>viable</u> tissue grafts precludes the application of a "sterilisation" technique to the tissue (as this would kill the tissue cells as well as the pathogens). Only mild "disinfection" techniques (e.g. antibiotic cocktails) can be applied, which reduces the sterility assurance of the graft.

As a result of these limitations to traditional tissue banking, more novel approaches have been evaluated in recent years. These have involved the manipulation of natural tissues or fabrication of tissue equivalents <u>in vitro</u> that will ideally either: -

1. Stimulate rapid tissue regeneration

or

2. Will immediately restore tissue function with the ability to self repair and grow and with a high degree of sterility assurance.

These approaches have been combined under the general heading of Tissue Engineering.

22.1 Tissue Engineered Materials that Stimulate Regeneration

In this case the implanted material is not intended to fulfil the functions of the missing, damaged, or diseased tissue; but rather to stimulate rapid regeneration of such tissue. This could include adding growth factors and cytokines to synthetic space filling materials to stimulate regeneration. However, these approaches are more commonly pursued by commercial companies, and is beyond the scope of this training manual. Emphasis here will be placed on the use of modified human tissues in tissue engineering. In this respect, one example of a regenerative tissue matrix is demineralised bone matrix. Bone comprises of a collagen protein matrix onto which the hard mineral component (hydroxyapatite) is deposited.

In addition, bound to the collagen component are a number of growth factors (cytokines, most of which belong to the TGFβ sub family) that are collectively known as bone morphogenetic proteins (BMPs). These signalling molecules are able to stimulate bone repair and regeneration. So for example, if a bone is fractured, this will expose some BMPs at the fracture surface, and these will in turn stimulate the "osteoclasts" and "osteoblasts" to begin to repair the fracture.

Advantage is taken of this natural process when de-mineralised bone matrix (DBM) powder is used. The donor bone is first ground into a powder or granules, and the mineral component is artificially dissolved away using hydrochloric acid. This leaves the collagen and BMPs now fully exposed. When the DBM is used clinically it rapidly stimulates bone regeneration.

Another strategy for stimulating regeneration that is being evaluated is the use of marrow derived stem cells. For example following a heart attack (myocardial infarct) some of the heart muscle is killed and fails to repair. It appears that the adjacent cardiac muscle cells do not have the capacity to regenerate new muscle. However, early studies have suggested that injection of bone marrow derived stem cells can lead to muscle regeneration. Further studies are underway to fully explore the potential of this method.

22.2 Tissue Engineered Materials that Functionally Replace Missing Tissue

The other area within "Tissue Banking" in which the principles of "Tissue Engineering" have been imported is in the modification of traditional tissue allografts to overcome some of the limitations alluded to in the introduction i.e. to develop a tissue graft that contains cells, or is rapidly colonised by recipient cells, without inducing acute allograft rejection responses. The objective being an analogue of an autograft i.e. a graft that will self repair and grow within the recipient.

One promising approach here has been to develop methods to remove allogeneic cells from an allograft without adversely affecting the biological and mechanical properties of the matrix. A number of decellularisation methods have been developed including the use of detergents, organic solvents and enzymes; or combinations of these treatments. Having removed the major immunostimulatory component it is expected that many tissues will then be re-colonised naturally in the recipient.

Where this still does not occur, an additional approach is to isolate appropriate cells from the recipient and to seed these into the cell-free allogeneic tissue matrix (for example see Figure 1). It is recognised that such composites may need to be validated in vitro prior to implantation and to this end bioreactors that simulate the in vivo biological and mechanical environment have been developed.

Significant advances with this approach to tissue replacement are expected in the next 5 to 10 year period.

<u>Examples</u>

(1) Decellularised Dermis
Decellularised dermis is a utility graft material that has been used in many different surgical indications; including correction of contour defects in dermis, hernia repair, as a sling to support internal organs and in shoulder (rotator cuff) injury as well as many others. The graft does become re-cellularised and is eventually re-modelled to become a functional graft within the recipient.

195

(2) Decellularised Heart Valves
Methods have been developed to decellularise heart valves to encourage recolonisation of the graft by recipient cells. Currently cryopreserved valves do not become recolonised and therefore do not self repair. Eventually the valves wear out and require replacement. In children, the cryopreserved valves fail to grow as the heart grows. This leads to size mismatch and the requirement to replace the valves with larger sized valves during development. There is significant morbidity and mortality associated with these repeat valve replacements. Again, the hope is that decellularised valves will become recolonised by the recipient's cells and hence be able to grow with the child. A recent study in Brazil indicated that the decellularised valves performed far better in patients than current cryopreserved valves with no failures at 4 years post-implantation. There were also indications that the recipient's cells were able to colonise the tissue matrix.

(3) Tissue Engineered Skin
As indicated in chapter 18, in order to provide a functional skin graft, an epidermis with a stratum corneum is necessary. This is unlikely to form fast enough if reliance is placed on a recolonisation process. Therefore in this case attempts have been made to recolonise the tissue matrix in vitro prior to grafting. Keratinocyte stem cells (progenitor cells) can be isolated from the epidermis of the recipient and greatly expanded in culture in vitro. Similarly, fibroblast cells from the dermis can also be expanded; and then both cell types seeded onto a decellularised dermal matrix of donor origin, according to the following method. It is hoped that this approach may ultimately produce viable skin grafts that will not be rejected.

Figure 1a. Tissue Engineering of Donor Skin

- Skin is de-epidermalised using the enzyme dispase (retains basement membrane intact).

- Dermal layer de-cellularised.

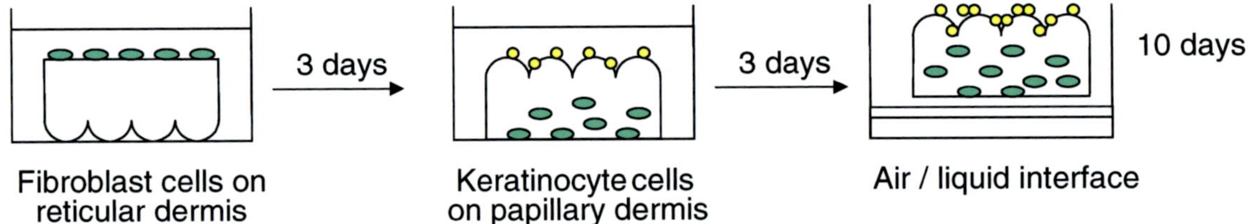

The skin is first de-cellularised by removing the epidermis entirely, and the cells within the dermis. The de-cellularised dermis is then inverted and seeded with the patient's (recipient's) fibroblasts. It is then turned to the correct orientation and patient-derived keratinocytes are seeded onto the basement membrane. It is raised to the air/liquid interface to allow normal keratinisation.

Figure 1b. Actual Histological Appearance of Fresh, De-cellularised and Re-Cellularised Skin

Fresh skin

De-cellularised, de-epidermalised dermal matrix

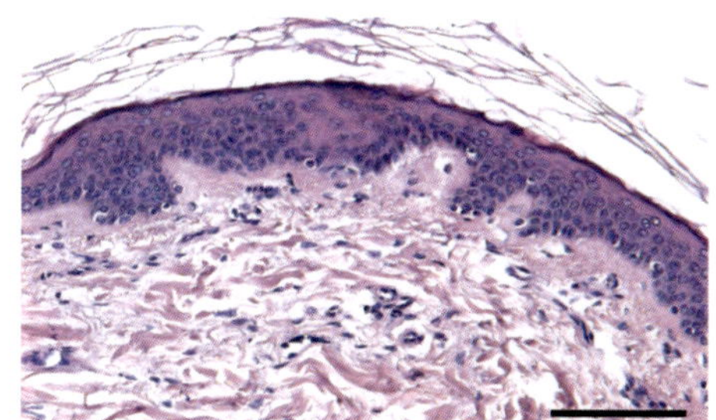

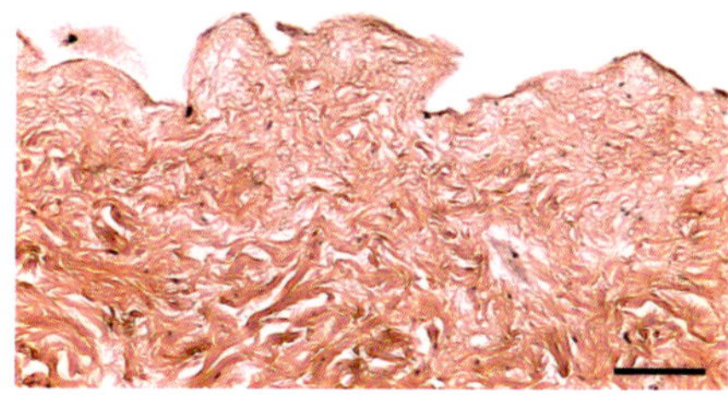

Re-cellularised skin

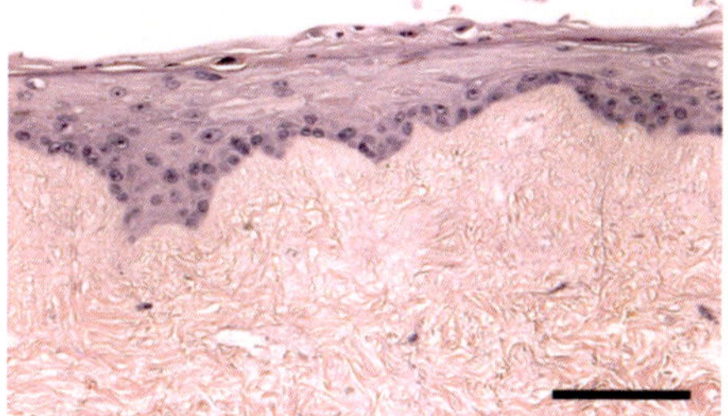

(4) Stem Cells

Whereas recipient skin is a tissue that is easily accessible and contains progenitor cells that can be used to populate decellularised donor tissue that is not the case for all tissues. For example, for specialist cardiac and vascular tissues, obtaining a biopsy to isolate progenitor cells could be highly dangerous.   An alternative approach would be to obtain stem cells from recipient bone marrow or other tissue sources (e.g. adipose tissue), and divert their differentiation along desired pathways to produce the progenitor cell types that are required.

22.3 Suggested Reading

1. Rowling PJ. et al. Fabrication and reorganisation of dermal equivalents suitable for skin grafting after major cutaneous injury. Biomaterials 11:181-185 (1990).
2. Kearney JN. Cryopreservation of cultured skin cells. Burns 17:380-383 (1991).
3. Daniels JT. et al. Human keratinocyte isolation and cell culture: a survey of current practices in the UK. Burns 22:35-39 (1996).
4. Daniels JT. et al. An investigation into the potential of extracellular matrix factors for attachment and proliferation of human keratinocytes on skin substitutes. Burns 23: 26-31 (1997).
5. Kearney JN et al. The osteoinductive properties of demineralised bone matrix grafts. Advances in Tissue Banking 1: 43-71 (1997).
6. Kearney J N. Clinical evaluation of skin substitutes. Burns 27:545-551 (2001).
7. Wilshaw S. et al. Production of an acellular amniotic membrane matrix for use in tissue engineering. Tissue Engineering, 12:2117-2129 (2006).
8. Kearney JN et al. Biocompatibility and recellularization potential of an acellular porcine heart valve matrix. Journal of Heart Valve Disease 14:228-237 (2005).
9. Francisco DA da Costa et al. Thirteen years experience with the Ross operation. The Journal of Heart Valve Disease 18:84-94 (2009.
10. Orlic, D et al. Bone marrow cells regenerate infarcted myocardium. Nature 410: 701-705 (2001).

22.4 Self Assessment Questions

Multiple Choice Questions

1. Donor tissues are rendered much less immunogenic by removing which one of the following?
   a) Collagen
   b) Cytokines
   c) Cells
   d) BMPs
   e) DNA

2. Which one of the following is a principle advantage expected of a tissue engineered product?
   a) Will last for up to 5 years
   b) Will perform better than natural tissue
   c) Restore tissue function and ability to self repair and grow
   d) Will be dependant on mechanical engineering
   e) Will be free of infectious agents

3. Which of the following are true?
   a) Osteoblasts are stem cells
   b) Osteoblasts are bone making cells
   c) Osteoclasts are bone making cells
   d) Osteocytes are bone making cells
   e) Osteoblasts belong to the macrophage cell family

4. Which of the following are true?
   a) Living grafts can be sterilised
   b) Living grafts can be disinfected with antibiotics
   c) The is no advantage in sterilising non-living grafts
   d) De-cellularised tissue cannot be sterilised
   e) De-cellularised tissue matrices can be sterilised

Short Answer Questions

1. What are BMPs and what do they do?
2. What are the disadvantages of using traditional banked tissues (viable or non-viable)?

Assignments

1. Compare the differing requirements of a tissue engineered skin graft from a tissue engineered heart valve graft.
2. Describe techniques used to de-cellularise tissue matrices.

23 ANSWERS TO SELF-ASSESSMENT QUESTIONS

Chapter 3. The Regulation of Cell and Tissue Banking

Multiple Choice Questions

1. b

2. b, c, d, e

3. a, b, c, d, e

4. a, b, d, e.

Short Answer Questions

The EU Tissue and Cells Directive covers the following key activities:
- Donation
- Procurement
- Testing
- Processing
- Preservation
- Storage
- Distribution of human tissue and cells.

The following cells and tissue are included:

- Haematopoietic peripheral blood cells, umbilical-cord (blood) and bone marrow stem cells
- Reproductive cells (eggs, sperm)
- Foetal tissues and cells
- Adult and embryonic stem cells
- Tissue

The following are excluded:
- Blood components
- organs

Question 2

Key points include:
- Premises and Equipment
  - Validated equipment (e.g. freezers)
  - Continuous temperature monitoring (24hours)
  - Licensed facility
  - Security

- Personnel
  - Appropriately qualified
  - Training and associated records

- Documentation
  - Standard Operating Procedures
  - Records (e.g. temperature monitoring, inventory, training records)

- Product
  - ➤ Packaging
  - ➤ Labelling
  - ➤ Temperature
  - ➤ Location
  - ➤ Expiry
  - ➤ Consent for storage
  - ➤ Traceability
  - ➤ Disposal arrangements

Chapter 4. The Collection, Use and Protection of Data

Multiple Choice Questions

1. e

2. c

3. e

4. e

Short Answer Questions

Question 1

Personal data, in written or electronic form must be:
- Fairly and lawfully processed;
- Processed for limited purposes;
- Adequate, relevant and not excessive for the purpose;
- Accurate;
- Kept no longer than necessary;
- Processed in accordance with the data subject's rights;
- Secure;
- Only transferred to countries with adequate data protection systems.

Question 2

These are the purposes which, according to the HT Act, generally require consent.

Purposes generally requiring consent where tissue is from living or deceased:
- Anatomical examination;
- Determining the cause of death (except where a post mortem is ordered by a coroner);
- Establishing after a person's death the efficacy of any drug or other treatment administered to them;
- Obtaining scientific or medical information (including genetic information) about a living or deceased person which may be relevant to any other person;
- Public display;
- Research in connection with disorders or the functioning of the human body;
- Transplantation

Purposes requiring consent when the tissue is from the deceased:

- Clinical audit;
- Education or training;
- Performance assessment;
- Public health monitoring;
- Quality assurance.

Chapter 5. Donor Screening and Testing

Multiple Choice Questions

1. b

2. d

3. a

4. d

Short Answer Questions

Question 1

Apart from the Hepatitis surface antigen test all the immunoassays rely on the development of anti-viral antibodies to test for the presence of the virus. This means that there is a window period from the time of initial infection to that of production of antibody. NAT testing reduces the window period for detecting the presence of the virus. This is particularly important for Hepatitis C which has a window period of 75 days when tested by conventional methods. NAT testing can reduce this to below 11 days.

Question 2

Haemodilution occurs when the blood within the body is diluted following the infusion with fluids (e.g. donor blood, plasma etc). This causes the blood sample taken from a deceased donor to be not representative of the serology status of that donor. A calculation must be done to ensure that the blood sample is representative. If not a blood sample must be found pre-haemodilution e.g. within a testing laboratory for cross matching.

Chapter 6. Aseptic Technique, Sterilisation, Irradiation, Disinfection and Quality Control for Tissues

Multiple Choice Questions

1. c

2. c

3. d

4. a

Short Answers

Question 1

Issues to consider include:
- Likelihood of contamination
- Level of contamination (bioburden)
- Pathogenicity of contaminants
- Adverse effects of decontamination on tissue properties

Question 2
Ethylene oxide is suitable for weight-bearing grafts.

Chapter 7. Cryopreservation

Multiple Choice Questions

1. c

2. b

3. a, b, c

4. c

Short Answer Questions

Question 1

Cooling rate controls the degree of intracellular supercooling which in turn controls the probability of intracellular freezing. It also controls the degree of exposure of the cells to raised solute concentrations at the higher temperatures where any chemical damage is greatest.

Chapter 8. Stem Cell Biology

Short Answer Questions

Question 1

A stem cell is a special kind of cell that has a unique capacity to renew itself and to give rise to defined cell types. A stem cell is uncommitted and remains uncommitted, until it receives a signal to develop into a specialised cell. Their proliferative capacity combined with the ability to become specialised makes stem cells unique.

Question 2

Sources of adult stem cells include bone marrow, blood, the cornea and the retina of the eye, brain, skeletal muscle, dental pulp, liver, skin, the lining of the gastrointestinal tract, and pancreas. The most abundant information about adult human stem cells comes from studies of haematopoietic stem cells isolated from the bone marrow and blood.

Chapter 9. Biology of Skin Tissue

Multiple Choice Questions

1. c, e

2. a, c

3. b

4. c, d

Short Answer Questions

Question 1

Advantages of living skin allografts include:
- Exhibits true graft take;
- Gains a blood supply;
- Buys time so, for example, a second crop of autografts can be taken.

Disadvantages of living skin allografts include:
- Will eventually be rejected;
- Cannot be sterilised.

Question 2

A thin (partial thickness) graft is taken from an area undamaged by the burn wound. This is transferred to an area of the (very deep or full thickness) burn wound. The graft takes and closes the wound.

Chapter 10. Biology of Musculo-Skeletal Tissue

Multiple Choice Questions

1. e

2. c

3. b

4. c

Short Answer Questions

Question 1

The five main functions of bone are:
- Support;
- Protection;
- Movement;
- Haemopoiesis;
- Mineral storage.

Question 2

Endochondral refers to the formation of a cartilage model first; intramembraneous refers to bone formation directly from mesenchyme. Endochondral is the major type and includes all long bones, intramembraneous occurs in flat bones - primarily the skull.

Chapter 11. Biology of Cardiovascular Tissue

Multiple Choice Questions

1. a, c

2. d

3. a

4. b

Short Answer Questions

Question 1

The mitral valve (also known as the bicuspid valve or left atrioventricular valve), is a dual flap (bi = 2) valve in the heart that lies between the left atrium (LA) and the left ventricle (LV).

Question 2

Viable donor cells in a heart valve graft are antigenic and so may lead to an increased immunogenic response against the graft.

Chapter 12. Biology and Processing of Ocular Tissue

Multiple Choice Questions

1. d

2. c

Short Answer Questions

Question 1

Solid tumours are usually acceptable in cornea donors because they metastasise (spread) via the blood circulation and the cornea is avascular. However, the use of sclera and limbal tissue is precluded in these patients because these tissues are vascularised.

Chapter 13. Haematopoietic Stem Cell Transplantation: An Overview

Multiple Choice Questions

1. b,c,d,e

2. a,b,c,d

3. a,d,e

4. a,b,d,e

Short Answer Questions

Question 1

Advantages:

- Higher proliferate potential than HPC, Apheresis and HPC, Marrow, therefore lower CD34 dose required.
- immunologically naive therefore lower risk of severe GvH
- A cord blood transplant can be performed with a 4 out of 6 HLA allele match (considering the HLA-A, -B, and -DRB1 genes), but ideally the unit should be matched for at least 5 out of 6 HLA alleles D. The tolerability of 2-HLA disparate grafts will likely increase the availability of HSC transplantation, particularly for patients with infrequent HLA haplotypes.
- double cord transplants enable cord transplantation option where single cords do not offer a sufficient dose
- directed cord blood collection is a possibility for sibling use
- could be useful for haematopoietic rescue following high dose therapy for non haematological malignancies
- in the future, autologous cord blood banked may be useful for regenerative medicine

Disadvantages:

- relapse in allogeneic cord blood transplantation is a possible limiting factor due to possible reduced graft vs. leukaemia effect although the literature is not conclusive on this point

- Delayed immune reconstitution post cord blood transplantation may mean greater susceptibility to infections

- Graft durability has been reported as lower than with HPC, Apheresis or HPC, Marrow

- small volumes with insufficient CD34 dose for adult recipients in particular

- unlikely to be useful for haematopoietic rescue following myeloablative treatment for haematological conditions cannot return to donor for more cells i.e. for donor lymphocytes

- Haematopoiesis is the process of production of blood and bone marrow cells.
- Pluripotent haematopoietic progenitor cells (HPC) or stem cells (HSCs) within bone marrow and give rise to all the cells of the haematopoietic system i.e. red cells, white cells and platelets.
- Pluripotent HPCs divide asymmetrically to yield another pluripotent daughter cell and a multipotent progenitor. Subsequent divisions of the latter ultimately give rise to cells which are committed to the various blood cell lineages.
- It is necessary to replenish stocks of pluripotent HSCs to maintain haematopoiesis during the entire lifespan.
- The process of haematopoiesis is regulated in health with a homeostatic balance maintained between numbers produced and those undergoing programmed cell death (apoptosis).
- The system is highly prolific and occurs in the proximal ends of the long bones, vertebral column, sternum and pelvic girdle in the adult.
- The bone marrow space is very vascular in areas of haematopoietic activity. This ensures an adequate supply of nutrients to the developing cells and a means to carry mature cells into the peripheral circulation.
- The stromal microenvironment in the bone marrow space provides support for the process of haematopoiesis. Developing HPCs are strongly adherent to the stomal cells during their development. Stromal cells secrete and also sequester molecules such as growth factors that support haematopoiesis.
- The system responds to positive and negative feedback influences depending on need i.e. haemorrhage will result in increased platelet and red blood production infection will result in increased white blood cell production.

Chapter 14. Collection of Haemopoietic Progenitor Cells (HPC)

Multiple Choice Questions

1. a, b, c, d
2. a, b
3. a, b

Short Answer Questions

Question 1

Following mobilisation with G-CSF with or without chemotherapy, vascular access enables blood to flow into and back from the apheresis machine. The machine centrifuges the incoming blood and separates buffy coat from red cell and plasma fractions. The mononuclear cell fraction contains the haematopoietic progenitor cells. Different apheresis technologies and different programmes will affect the volume, concentration, speed and reliability of peripheral blood stem cell collections.

Question 2

G-CSF with or without chemotherapy is given 5 to 7 days prior to the estimated date of harvest. The patient's underlying condition, conditioning chemotherapy, the timing and dose of G-CSF all affect the prediction of the harvest date but this is often imprecise. Peripheral blood taken from the donor or patient prior to harvest and assayed for total white count, MNC and CD34+ concentrations will inform on the best harvest date. There is a close correlation between the peripheral blood CD34+ concentration and the yield of CD34+ cells.

Chapter 15. Processing and Quality Control of Haematopoietic Stem Cells for Transplantation

Multiple Choice Questions

1. b, c
2. a, d
3. d
4. c, d

Short Answer Questions

Question 1

This device is used for making aseptic connections. The two lines of PVC tubing that need to be joined (A and B) are clamped in a parallel configuration in the device. Single-use copper wafers are heated by the device to 320°C. The wafer cuts each piece of tubing into two and then the tubing sections are moved along the heated wafer and re-aligned such that B1 is brought adjacent to A2. The wafer is lowered and the device welds the two cut ends together and holds them in position until the joint is cool enough to be handled. The temperature of the wafer is sufficient to ensure sterility is maintained.

Question 2

The CliniMACS is a computer controlled device, which incorporates a permanent magnet, a peristaltic pump and pinch valves. A sterile tubing set is installed in the device with a separation column containing a ferro-magnetic matrix inserted into the path of the magnet. CD34+ cells labelled with antibody chemically coupled to super paramagnetic particles are retained by the magnet allowing the T cell rich fraction to pass into a collection bag. Following washing of the retained CD34+ve cells these are eluted from the magnet into a separate product bag. The CliniMACS is capable of 4-5 log depletion of T cells in the product compared to the starting material.

Chapter 16. Cord Blood Banking

Multiple Choice Questions

1. a, c, d, e
2. a, b, c, d, e
3. e
4. a, b, d, e

Short Answer Questions

Question 1

The larger the cord blood collection the more likely it is to contain higher numbers of nucleated cells and haematopoietic stem cells. These units are ultimately more likely to be successful in transplantation than units containing smaller numbers of stem cells and can provide for larger patients.

Where the donor mother went, when and how long for. Record the details of all countries visited with dates, including stopovers, to determine visitor status. This information is needed to assess whether further testing is required of the donor mother to exclude the risk of infections such as malaria or Trypanosomiasis cruzi.

Chapter 17. Histocompatibility & Immunogenetics of Transplantation

Multiple Choice Questions

1. b,c,d,e
2. a,b,c,d
3. a,d,e
4. a,b,d,e

Short Answer Questions

Question 1

A method for amplification of small fragments of DNA using a heat-stable DNA polymerase. It works through a chain reaction of three stages repeated between 20 to 40 times.

Heat to >94°C. Causes denaturation of DNA where the strands of DNA separate to form single-stranded DNA.

Cool to 60 - 65°C. Allows binding of single-stranded oligonucleotides, known as 'primers'. The selection of the primer sites are critical to ensure specificity. Primers are designed and manufactured with complementary sequences to give optimal annealing at 60 to 62°C.

Heat to 72°C. Allows extension of the primers along the complementary DNA strands by Taq polymerase.

Automated cycling of these stages in thermal cyclers allows exponential expansion of the selected DNA region. Thirty cycles takes about 45 minutes and amplified DNA (amplicons) can be visualised by electropheresis using agarose or polyacrylamide gels.

Question 2

HLA reactive antibodies may occur following exposure to HLA antigens in pregnancy, following red cell or platelet transfusion or transplantation. The degree of HLA matching required for allogeneic stem cell transplantation is high so the risk from HLA-reactive antibodies is relatively low. When they do occur, their significance will depend on titre and specificity; antibody titres are usually low, and their titre will generally fall following myeloablative treatment. Residual antibodies in the recipient are generally adsorbed onto donor cells infused with the graft. However, HLA antibodies to antigens expressed at high levels on T cells may contribute to T cell depletion following transplantation.

Chapter 18. Transfusion of Stem Cell Transplant Patients

Multiple Choice Questions

1. a, b, d

2. a, d, e

3. c

4. d

Short Answer Questions

Question 1

Platelets are given when platelet count is less than 10 in stable thrombocytopenic patients, when less than 20 if there is fever or other factors associated with non-immune platelet consumption and less than 50 if interventions are performed. Measure platelet count daily.

Question 2

Transfer of immunocompetent B lymphocytes in the graft which recognise A, B antigens in the patient and produce anti-A, B. Treatment with CAMPATH antibodies and CD34+ cell selection prevent immune mediated haemolysis post-BMT (passenger lymphocyte syndrome). Selective T cell depletion does not prevent this condition.

Chapter 19. Collection and Retrieval of Tissue

Multiple Choice Questions

1. c

2. c, d

3. a, d

4. a, b, c

Short Answer Questions

Question 1

A physical examination is performed to determine donor suitability according to current standards/legislation. Findings may indicate high behaviour risk or indicate signs of infection which can lead to rejection of the donor.

Examples include (but are not limited to):
- Old/new intravenous drug sites (non-medical)/track marks
- Unknown Tattoos (possibly covering track marks)
- Unexplained jaundice
- Unknown piercings
- Swellings/bruising
- Skin redness

3 points of identification are required. Examples include (but are not limited to):

ID of choice:
- Full name (first/last name);
- Date of birth;
- Address;
- Hospital number.

Only 1 item to be used for ID purposes from the below list:
- Donation of corneas (eyes);
- Specific identifiable tattoos;
- Specific identifiable distinguishing marks e.g. birth mark, scarring;
- Specific identifiable jewellery;
- Written/verbal confirmation from a Health Care Professional (e.g. mortuary technician, Coroner etc);
- Circumstances of death.

Chapter 20. Tissue Processing, Storage and Issue

Multiple Choice Questions

1. b

2. d

3. b

4. d

3. c

5. a

Short Answers

Question 1

- Removal of marrow has been shown to increase the rate of incorporation.
- There is a possibility that disease causing agents could be present in bone marrow.
- To permit storage at room temperature following lyophilisation.
- To improve the cosmetic appearance of the graft.

Question 2

Tendons are decontaminated to remove the requirement for terminal sterilisation. They are decontaminated through treatment with chemicals such as ethanol.

Question 3

The cleaning protocol, routinely applied before excision of corneoscleral discs, reduces the microbial load on the ocular surface. Antibiotics and antimycotics in the organ culture medium are highly effective in minimising microbiological load in the higher (34-37C) storage temperature. These combined with the length of incubation (storage up to 28 days) and monitoring of the storage medium allow the tissue to be kept safe for the clinical use.

Chapter 21. Clinical Aspects of Tissue Transplantation

Multiple Choice Questions

1. b

2. c

3. d

4. d

Short Answer Questions

Question 1

Advantages of cryopreserved human heart valves include:
- Low incidence of calcification and infection;
- Reduced chances of reoperation;
- Long term anticoagulation therapy is not required.

Question 2

Risks include:
- Transmission of viruses and infections;
- Bacterial and fungal contamination.

Prevention measures include:
- Donor selection using guidelines;
- Testing;
- Aseptic retrieval techniques;
- Validated processing methods (GMP);
- Screening products for contamination;
- Terminal sterilisation if required;
- Washing to remove marrow for vCJD risk reduction;
- Limiting donor exposure.

Chapter 22. Tissue Engineering

Multiple Choice Questions

1. c

2. c

3. b

4. b, d

Short Answer Questions

Question 1

Bone morphogenetic proteins (BMPs) are cytokines/growth factors that induce rapid bone regeneration. They induce mesenchymal stem cells to differentiate into osteoblasts and begin bone formation. After numerous animal studies using BMP, it was used for the first time in 1997 in a clinical trial of patients undergoing spinal fusion. 10 of the 11 patients enrolled in the study had successful fusions within 3 months of surgery, all without the unpleasant side effects of bone grafting

Disadvantages of traditionally banked tissues include:
- May not be incorporated/recolonised by recipient cells;
- May not grow;
- May not self repair;
- Viable grafts may be rejected;
- Viable grafts cannot be sterilised.

24 ABBREVIATIONS AND TERMINOLOGY

7-AAD	7-aminoactinomycin D
ACL	Anterior cruciate ligament
AMT	Amniotic membrane transplant
APC	Antigen presenting cell
ATC	Anti-thymocyte globulin
ATD	Adult therapeutic dose
BATB	British Association for Tissue Banking
BBMR	British Bone Marrow Registry
BBTS	British Blood Transfusion Society
BC	Buffy coat
BM	Bone marrow
BMP	Bone morphogenetic protein
BMT	Bone marrow transplant
BSE	Bovine spongiform encephalopathy
CB	Cord blood
CBB	Cord blood bank
CEA	Cultured epithelial autograft
CFUGM	Colony forming unit granulocyte macrophage
CI	Count increment
CJD	Creutzfeldt-Jakob disease
CLP	Common lymphoid progenitor
CML	Chronic myeloid leukaemia
CMP	Common myeloid progenitor
CMV	Cytomegalovirus
CyA	Cyclosporin A
DBM	De-mineralised bone matrix
DC	Dendritic cell
DIC	Disseminated intravascular coagulation
DLI	Donor lymphocyte infusion
DMSO	Dimethyl sulphoxide
EBMT	European Group for Blood and Marrow Transplantation
EBV	Epstein Barr virus
ERH	Equilibrium relative humidity
ESC	Embryonic stem cell
FACT	Foundation for Accreditation of Cellular Therapy
FBC	Full blood count

FFP	Fresh frozen plasma
FITC	Fluorescein isothiocyanate
FNHTR	Febrile non-haemolytic transfusion reaction
G-CSF	Granulocyte-colony stimulating factor
GMP	Good manufacturing practice
GvHD	Graft versus host disease
GvL	Graft versus leukaemia
H&I	Histocompatibility and Immunogenetics
HBV	Hepatitis B virus
HCV	Hepatitis C virus
HIV	Human Immunodeficiency Virus
HPC, Apheresis	Haematopoietic progenitor cell – apheresis
HPC, Cord Blood	Haematopoietic progenitor cell – cord blood
HPC, Marrow	Haematopoietic progenitor cell – bone marrow
HSC	Haematopoietic stem cell
HSCT	Haematopoietic stem cell transplant
HTA	Human Tissue Authority
HTLV	Human T Lymphotropic Virus
IEF	Isoelectric focusing
ISCT	International Society for Cell Therapy
JACIE	Joint Accreditation Committee of ISCT-Europe and EBMT
JPAC	Joint UKBTS/NIBSC Professional Advisory Committee
LCM	Leukocyte-conditioned medium
Mab	Monoclonal antibody
MAPC	Multipotent adult progenitor cell
MHRA	Medicines and Healthcare products Regulatory Agency
MK	McCarey-Kaufman medium
MLR	Mixed lymphocyte reaction
MSBT	Committee on the Microbiological Safety of Blood and Tissues for Transplantation
MSC	Mesenchymal stem cell
NAT	Nucleic acid amplification technology
NHSBT	National Health Service Blood and Transplant
NIBSC	National Institute of Biological Standards and Control
NK	Natural killer
PCL	Posterior cruciate ligament
PCR	Polymerase chain reaction
PCV	Packed cell volume

PE	Phycoerythrin
PK	Penetrating keratoplasty
PRP	Platelet rich plasma
PT	Prothombin time
QA	Quality Assurance
QC	Quality Control
RBC	Red blood cell
RIC	Reduced intensity conditioning
SAC	Standing Advisory Committee
SAL	Sterility assurance level
SBT	Sequence-based typing
SCID	Severe combined immunodeficiency
SCR	SCID repopulating cells
SOP	Standard Operating Procedure
SSOP	Sequence specific oligonucleotide probe
SSP	Sequence specific primer
STR	Short tandem repeat analysis
TBI	Total body irradiation
TC-T Cells	T Cells Therapeutic. Therapeutic cell product containing quantified T cell population
TEP	Tissue engineered product
TNC	Total nucleated cells
TRALI	Transfusion-related acute lung injury
TRM	Transplant-related mortality
TSE	Transmissible spongiform encephalopathy
TTI	Transfusion transmitted infection
TTP	Thrombotic thrombocytopenic purpura
VUD	Unrelated volunteer donor